Naturalistic Observation

Michael V. Angrosino

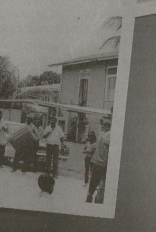

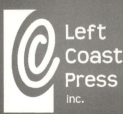

Left Coast Press inc.

Walnut Creek, CA

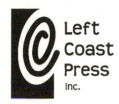

1630 North Main Street, #400
Walnut Creek, CA 94596
http://www.LCoastPress.com
Copyright © 2007 by Left Coast Press, Inc.

All rights reserved. No part of this publication may be reproduced stored in a retrieval system, or transmitted in any form or by any means, electronic, mechanical, photocopying, recording, or otherwise, without the prior permission of the publisher.

Library of Congress Cataloging-in-Publication Data

Angrosino, Michael V.

Naturalistic observation / Michael V. Angrosino.

p. cm. -- (Qualitative essentials)

Includes bibliographical references.

ISBN-13: 978-1-59874-059-2 (hardback : alk. paper)

ISBN-10: 1-59874-059-8 (hardback : alk. paper)

ISBN-13: 978-1-59874-060-8 (pbk. : alk. paper)

ISBN-10: 1-59874-060-1 (pbk. : alk. paper)

1. Ethnology--Methodology. 2. Ethnology--Research. I. Title.

GN345.A56 2007

305.8001--dc22

Printed in the United States of America

The paper used in this publication meets the minimum requirements of American National Standard for Information Sciences—Permanence of Paper for Printed Library Materials, ANSI/NISO Z39.48–1992.

Edited by Megan Pearson
Designed by Murray Pearson
Email editing@autographic.ca for more information.

07 08 09 10 11   5 4 3 2 1

Contents

Acknowledgements

I am grateful to Mitch Allen of Left Coast Press, Inc., and to Janice Morse, the general editor of this series for giving me the opportunity to share my enthusiasm for qualitative research in general and for observational techniques in particular. Their very astute and helpful comments kept me on track throughout the process of writing and revising this manuscript.

I also acknowledge my students at the University of South Florida who have engaged me in creative dialogue about qualitative methods over the years and whose needs as budding researchers have shaped my approach to this topic. I also once again thank Petra LeClair for incomparable clerical and editorial assistance.

The photos in this book were taken over the course of several ethnographic visits to Trinidad in the West Indies. Most of them are over thirty years old. As such they predate the current era of informed consent that is discussed in the chapter on ethics, although all the people in the pictures gave me general verbal consent to use their images "for purposes of research." I thank them for their willingness to share their lives with me and, by extension, with the readers of this book.

— Michael V. Angrosino

Chapter One

What Is Naturalistic Observation?

What is Naturalistic Observation?

Qualitative research is a process of inquiry aimed at understanding human behavior by building complex, holistic pictures of the social and cultural settings in which such behavior occurs. It does so by analyzing words rather than numbers, and by reporting the detailed views of the people who have been studied. Such inquiry is conducted in settings where people naturally interact, as opposed to specially designed laboratories or clinical/experimental settings. Qualitative research seeks to understand the what, how, when, and where of an event or an action in order to establish its meanings, concepts, definitions, characteristics, metaphors, symbols, and descriptions (Berg, 2004, pp. 2–3; Creswell, 1998, pp. 14–16).

Prominent among the tools of qualitative research is **observation,** characterized by Adler and Adler (1994) as "the fundamental base of all research methods" (p. 389). Quantitative researchers favor observing people in highly controlled settings in which the researchers control all the variables involved, with the aim of experimentally testing specific hypotheses. By contrast, qualitative researchers use observation as a process by which people interacting in their natural settings are studied so that their behaviors and words can be put into their proper context. The descriptive study of people in their natural settings is sometimes referred to as **ethnography** or ethnographic research. Although hypotheses may be derived from naturalistic observations, the observations themselves do not usually arise from a hypothesis-testing model of research. Qualitative researchers may refer to the natural settings where their projects are conducted as "the field," and when they leave the laboratory to do their research, they are said to be conducting **fieldwork**.

It should be emphasized from the outset that naturalistic observation as a tool of research is different from the kinds of casual "seeing" that we do in the course of everyday life, even if it in fact stems from those very ordinary life skills. In order to be useful for research, observation must be **systematic**, which means that it must be conducted carefully, with precise notation that allows for the efficient and orderly retrieval, categorization, and analysis of information (Adler and Adler, 1994). While qualitative researchers tend to avoid predetermining categories of action that can be precisely measured, they are as concerned as their quantitative colleagues with ensuring that observation yields more than haphazard impressions. In everyday language, "observation" usually refers to the use of our visual sense to record and make

sense of information. But in the research context, we must learn to use all of our senses, in order to accurately perceive the whole picture. As Adler and Adler (1994, p. 378) put it, "Observation thus consists of gathering impressions of the surrounding world through all relevant human faculties."

There are three main traditions of observation-based research within qualitative social science: the **non-reactive** (or **unobtrusive**) mode, in which the researcher avoids intervening in the action he or she is observing, the **reactive** mode, in which the researcher intervenes in the action, but only in the role of outside observer, and the **participant** mode, in which the researcher strives to be an active member of the group under study. There are important sub-divisions of these three broad categories that we will discuss in greater detail in a later section. At this point, however, we can say that all forms of qualitative observation-based inquiry are rooted in the researcher's preference for the "natural laboratory." It is assumed that observation of people and events takes place in the settings in which they would naturally occur, and involves those who would naturally take part in them. The aim of qualitative observation research is to capture the essential flow of everyday experience. As such, observation serves the purpose of detecting patterns, concepts, trends, or categories that are taken as meaningful by people in the course of that everyday experience; it does not begin, as does much quantitative inquiry, with patterns, concepts, trends, or categories that emerge from theoretical formulations and take the form of specific hypotheses that can be tested by measuring clearly operationalized variables.

Adler and Adler (1994, p. 378), for example, speak of the "'Click!' experience," which they describe as "a sudden, though minor, epiphany as to the emotional depth or importance of an event or a phenomenon." Real life, in other words, is full of surprises, even for the well trained and experienced researcher. Observation allows the researcher to register that surprise and then ponder the meaning behind the behavior that provoked it. It is my belief that this necessary element of surprise and the experience of epiphany best arise out of personal encounters; it is fine to read about the research of others, but doing research for oneself is the best way to learn ethnography. Therefore, in addition to the didactic presentations in the following chapters, this book will feature some do-it-yourself suggestions. Those labeled "For Discussion" are meant to stimulate thinking about the research process and are intended to be shared with some relevant peer group.

Why Do Qualitative Researchers Choose Naturalistic Observation as a Research Tool?

As we will see, good fieldwork is usually a matter of putting together multiple data collection techniques so as to converge on a holistic picture of a setting. Observation is rarely conducted in isolation as the sole method of data collection. In the context, then, of a mixed-methods research project, we can say that observational techniques are particularly well-suited to getting the lay of the land, so to speak. Observations therefore form the basis from which we can develop questions for surveys or interviews. In that sense, they are essential to and inform all other forms of data collection in the field. Using observation to get the lay of the land typically involves the study of:

- specific settings that may be clearly demarcated in physical space (e.g., a shopping mall, a church, a school) or in virtual space (e.g., an on-line chat group)

- events that feature well-defined sequences of activities longer and more complex than single actions, that take place in specific locations, have a defined purpose and meaning, involve more than one person, have a recognized history, and are repeated with some regularity (e.g., a university commencement program)

- demographic factors, which might include, for example, observation of housing or building materials, presence or absence of indoor plumbing, presence and number of intact windows, methods of garbage disposal, and legal or illegal sources of electrical power to indicate socioeconomic differences between neighborhoods as well as observations of where people congregate under particular circumstances.

Site Selection: Examples

The first step in a naturalistic observation inquiry is to select a site in which to conduct fieldwork. In principle, qualitative observation-based research can be conducted wherever people interact in "natural" settings. The method originally came into its own in the context of research in small-scale and relatively homogeneous communities, although it soon came to be used in well-defined enclave communities (defined by race, ethnicity, or social class) within larger societies. More recently, it has been applied to "communities of interest," defined as groups of people who share some common factor, such as members of a support group for cancer survivors, who do not necessarily share all the other aspects of traditional culture beyond the one interest that brought them together. It has even begun to be applied to "virtual communities" formed in cyberspace rather than in traditional physical space. In the latter case, there may be legitimate questions raised about whether all the senses are truly engaged in the process of observation, but an adaptation of the method is almost certainly called for, given the propensity of people nowadays to spend proportionately greater amounts of their time interacting on-line.

Public spaces and opportunity-based site selection.

An observational research site may be one in which the researcher might find him/herself anyway and which is considered "public" in a way that requires no special access; observations in **public space** have taken place in airports, city streets, shopping malls, medical waiting areas, and sporting events. On the other hand, a site may be one which the researcher might need permission to enter: a school classroom, a private event like a wedding or a funeral, or certain places of worship. It is conceivable that a site may not be "chosen" at all, but may present itself to the researcher through happenstance. Some years ago at an unusually long commencement ceremony, I amused myself by making note of facial expressions and body language that seemed to differentiate faculty from students as we progressed (at a glacial pace) through the event. I even wrote a paper about my observations, although the explicit threat of cruel reprisals from my colleagues kept me from ever publishing it.

Site selection for theoretical interests.

More often than not, however, a site is specifically selected for some definite purpose (albeit typically not a formally stated, testable hypothesis). A site might be selected because the researcher has a prior theoretical interest in a particular aspect of sociocultural behavior that is typically found at such a site. One of my research interests, for example, is the way in which ethnic groups in culturally diverse societies define their communal identities, and how those identities shift in response to evolving economic and political circumstances. A study I conducted on Trinidad, an island in the West Indies, dealt specifically with how people from India (brought to the island in colonial times on a system of indenture to work on sugar plantations following the emancipation of the slaves) had made the transition from being an impoverished rural proletariat to being part of the emerging national state. During the course of this research, I conducted on-site observations at both a traditional sugar mill in the countryside and a modern oil refinery near the international port. I was not particularly concerned with the physics and chemistry of the transformation of cane into molasses or of petroleum into gasoline, but rather in the kinds of social interaction that typified the mill, an almost exclusively Indian work site, in comparison to the refinery, where Indians worked in close proximity to people from many different ethnic groups. (See Angrosino, 1974.)

Site selection for policy issues.

A site might also be selected because it typifies an **issue of current policy** concern. My own long-term study of adults with mental "disabilities" derived initially from my skeptical reaction to a spate of alarmist news reports about the "epidemic" of homeless mentally ill people who were "flooding" the streets in the wake of the mass closing of mental institutions. I wanted to get beyond the sensationalized media accounts in order to understand the process of deinstitutionalization from the inside, and so I began observing sheltered workshops, group homes, training centers, and other sites at which deinstitutionalized adults labeled as mentally retarded and/or chronically mentally ill congregated. (See Angrosino, 1998a.)

Site selection for a research commission.

Another way in which a site may become the focus of observational research is through a process of **commissioning, paid or otherwise**. That is, the people or organization involved in that site may want to have research conducted, and will contract with someone for this purpose.

For example, a nearby monastery was getting ready to celebrate the centennial of its founding, and its leaders thought that an article on daily life in the community would make an interesting addition to the series of publications being released to celebrate the event. Since the study of the role of religious institutions in secular society is another of my interests, I have developed contacts with members of various denominations in our area. Through those contacts I was brought to the attention of the abbot of the monastery, who asked me to conduct the research he had in mind. Although much of my study was based on interviews with the monks, I was only able to place their reminiscences in proper context by doing a thorough observation of the site and getting a feel for what living there would be like. (See Angrosino, 2004.) The monastery "commission" was undertaken as an act of community service— assisting a significant local institution in celebrating an important anniversary. I have, however, conducted other research projects for which remuneration was offered; those projects usually involved program evaluation and/or needs assessments of programs offering services to people with disabilities. Most agencies that accept public funding of one sort or another require such studies as part of their official records, in order to demonstrate their public accountability.

Site selection for research linkage.

Sometimes a site is opened up for observation because it is linked with another site in which research is already being conducted. One aspect of my interest in religion in secular society is a comparative study of hospital chaplaincy programs (Angrosino, 2006). An important function of chaplains in many hospitals is ministry in emergency rooms and trauma centers. Since I was already accepted as part of the pastoral care teams at the several hospitals I was studying, I had entrée into their ERs—something that would have been difficult had I approached the hospital administrators on my own, without prior involvement, solely on the basis of my theoretical interest in the issue. In any case, I am now in the midst of a more systematic observation of interaction among the various categories of professionals at work in the ER setting. This sort of site selection is sometimes referred to as "opportunistic" because it comes from a willingness to take advantage of opportunities that arise spontaneously; the word, however, has negative connotations in ordinary discourse, and some scholars prefer to avoid it when discussing research.

Basic Principles of Site Selection

We may summarize the basic principles of site selection as follows:

Select a site so that the issue (be it academic/theoretical or of a current-events nature) can be studied in a reasonably clear fashion.

My interest in the evolution of ethnic identity, as illustrated by migrants from India to the Western Hemisphere, could have been conducted in any number of sites with significant Indian populations. But some of those places, such as Suriname on the north coast of South America, were quite isolated at the time of my initial study, and therefore had Indian populations that had scarcely begun the process of assimilation. There were also communities of West Indian Indians in large urban centers in North America (e.g., New York, Toronto), but they had already completed most of the process. Trinidad seemed to be a good compromise, as its Indian community was neither too traditional nor already too assimilated. Similarly, a study of the effects of deinstitutionalization required a site that had sufficient numbers of adults with mental retardation, that is, a place where such people were likely to seek jobs, housing, and so forth. A rural community with a lone mentally challenged individual would not have been a reasonable site.

Select a site that is comparable to others that have been studied by other researchers, but not one that has itself been over-studied. People in communities with the misfortune of being located near a university campus may well feel that they have been studied to the point of exhaustion; even the best intentioned and most hospitable people reach a point where they feel they have answered the same questions one too many times. (There is an old joke among anthropologists to the effect that the typical Navajo family consists of a mother, a father, three children, and an anthropologist.) On the other hand, it is not necessary to go off to the far corners of the planet in order to find a community that is untouched insofar as research is concerned. Once again, striking an appropriate balance is of the utmost importance. For example, my deinstitutionalization study was inspired by research conducted by colleagues in California; my own observations took me to Florida, Tennessee, Indiana, and the Washington DC area—comparable situations, but with their own distinctive social and political attributes, and ones that had not yet been studied to the same extent as in California. Similarly, I was aware of numerous studies of overseas Indian communities in Africa and the Pacific, as

well as in the Caribbean; there had even been several in Trinidad. But as most of the research on Trinidad had been conducted in the traditional sugar cane-growing areas, I deliberately set out to find a village that was in transition from agrarian life to one oriented toward employment at the oil refinery.

Select a site in which the research will not come to be seen as a burden on the local population.

Researchers can overstay their welcome and become nuisances in many ways beyond merely being too obtrusive in their observational techniques. If they are living in the community, they must be conscious of the possibility that they are imposing on the hospitality of their hosts, as well as draining their resources. A contemporary monastery is heir to a centuries-long tradition of hospitality and is set up to accommodate visitors. A typical village in Trinidad, by contrast, receives few outside visitors and does not have guest houses, restaurants, or other tourist amenities, which means that the researcher must live in a family's home and accommodate himself to their routines and practices. The researcher also needs to be conscious of the fact that the family is likely not very affluent by U.S. standards, and that regardless of how welcoming they might be they cannot be expected to provide for all their guest's needs without some compensation. While researchers may indeed welcome an invitation to reciprocity, they may not be prepared for what the community considers appropriate repayment for bearing the burdens of the research project. Some researchers dislike making monetary compensation for research support, not because they are cheapskates, but because their cultural values suggest that a relationship based on monetary exchange can be impersonal, impeding the kind of intimate participation that many fieldworkers seek. One certainly does not want to be in the position of buying cooperation, but there is nothing inherently wrong with offering to defray the costs of goods and services, such as room and board, which obviously are added expenses on already tight budgets. Compensation can also be non-monetary; different settings will exhibit their own norms about what does and does not constitute appropriate reciprocity among friends.

Gaining Entrée

Observations conducted in public space can commence as soon as the researcher arrives on the scene. Sites that are more restricted do, however, require some form of permission before research can begin.

Informal gatekeepers.

In general, people who control access to a research site are known as "gatekeepers." In many cases, entrée may be gained through relatively informal means, especially when the gatekeepers are insiders who agree to introduce researchers to the community and vouch for their trustworthiness and for the value of the proposed research. Researchers do well, however, to ensure that such informal gatekeepers really are individuals who are trusted by the community; it sometimes happens that people who put themselves forward to play such a role are, in fact, marginal to the community, and are using the proposed research as a way of either enhancing their own status or of advancing a personal agenda. Associating oneself with such dubious characters does nothing to promote the efficient work of the researcher. Wilson (1974), for example, describes in amusing detail his capture by an eccentric character who presented himself as a leader of a small Caribbean island but who turned out to be considered a madman by the rest of the people.

Formal gatekeepers.

In some settings, entrée may require dealing with more formally constituted gatekeeping; clearances from police or other officials may be required in writing. In such circumstances, researchers should keep in mind that while having official sanction may be desirable, and even necessary, it might also have the drawback of identifying the research project to those in charge— which might not endear researchers to the rest of the community, depending on the nature of local politics and social interactions. It should be noted that gaining entrée is not always a one-shot deal but rather a continuing series of negotiations. In the days when cultural anthropologists in particular conceived of research as lasting for at least a year in one site, this process of negotiation became part of the fabric of research itself. In shorter term research, which is more common today, the process must be consciously speeded up.

How Researchers
Position Themselves in the Field

We will devote a separate section to the ethics of research—the obligations researchers owe to the people they study. But a word needs to be said here about researchers' obligations to themselves. In all forms of qualitative research, the researcher is the primary instrument of research—one human being interacting (to one degree or another) with other human beings. It is, therefore, most important to know yourself before committing to any research site. It should be clear that certain sites might be unacceptable on personal grounds, even if they are appropriate to the project in terms of theory, current events, and so forth. For example, researchers who do not want to witness scenes of physical suffering would probably not care to observe an ER, no matter how much doing so might further the understanding of an issue of theoretical or policy concern. People who have personal issues with organized religion would probably need to work extra hard to set aside their preconceptions when observing a community, such as a monastery, explicitly set up for religious purposes. Researchers who are uneasy in situations of conflict might want to avoid working in communities that are polarized or factionalized in some way. Most people would probably consciously avoid putting themselves in situations involving criminal activity; even if they do not object to something that is technically illegal (e.g., they are politically sympathetic to undocumented migrants) they might not want to be put in a compromising position of knowing about—and feeling pressured to inform about—those illegal activities. And they might be very reluctant to place themselves in situations of real and immediate danger (war zones, high crime neighborhoods). It should be said that researchers can and do work in all of these situations. The point, however, is to decide where one draws the line defining one's personal comfort zone. While it is good to challenge oneself and go outside that zone, no research is worth making oneself *so* uncomfortable that the quality of the resulting data is questionable.

Necessary Research Skills

In addition to defining and maintaining an appropriate degree of comfort in the research setting, researchers should also refine the following basic skills and attributes in order to be able to conduct observational research with maximum efficiency:

- **Language facility**: The ability to pick up on nuances of expression, keeping in mind that people communicate through gestures, body language, and the use of space in addition to what they say in words.

- **Explicit awareness**: The ability to perceive the mundane details that most people filter out of their routine observations)

- **Good memory**: It's not always possible to record observations on the spot.

- **Cultivated naiveté**: Never being afraid to ask the obvious question.

- **Writing facility**: in the final analysis, most observational data will only be useful when placed in some sort of narrative context)

Researchers contemplating an observational study might do well to begin with a candid self-assessment, stressing the following points: their emotional and attitudinal state; their physical and mental health (and the health of anyone who might be a companion or associate in the research process); their areas of competence and incompetence; and their ability to set aside preconceptions about people, behaviors, or socio-political situations. There are some personal factors that can be relatively easy to modify so that an observer can fit into a study community more readily. For example, hair styles, types of jewelry or body adornments, clothing, or tone of voice can all generate cues for people at the site to respond to, whether positively or negatively. But there are some factors that are beyond our control: for example, one's age, gender, or perceived racial or ethnic category. It is therefore important to consider the degree to which these qualities might affect the role of the observer at the site. If they represent barriers too difficult to overcome, another site should be selected, as researchers should never become objects of attention to such a degree that the objectives of their research are overshadowed. Matters pertaining to researchers' identities (both the way they see themselves and the way they are perceived by others) and their impact on the conduct of fieldwork will be discussed in greater detail in a later section.

Necessary Interpersonal and Social Skills

There are some additional factors that should be kept in mind when considering ways in which to gain entrée into a community:

- **Researchers should not assume that communities similar to their own will be easier to work with, and easier to fit into.**

It is sometimes the case that the more researchers are like the people they are studying, the more the latter will expect of them and the less tolerant they are likely to be of the insistence on doing research rather than just hanging out all the time. Sometimes researchers who are obviously outsiders are able to do better research because people in the community will understand that they really do need help figuring out what is going on. It is certainly true that researchers have an important head start when working in communities similar to their own, but there is also the danger that they will take too much for granted and will not be sufficiently careful in recording and analyzing the minute details of behavior that is overly familiar to them.

- **Researchers should make every effort to be helpful to the community; they should not be seen as those who only take, but never give.**

What is given, however (material compensation, doing favors of one sort or another) is dependent on the circumstances of both the researchers and the study communities. It is both unwise and unethical to promise assistance as a means of gaining entrée even though it will clearly be impossible to follow through on the agreement.

- **Researchers should take the time to explain their purposes—a matter that will be treated in greater detail in the section on ethics below.**

Researchers working in teams should make sure that the community is ready and willing to accommodate everyone, and that each member of the team—not just the principal investigator on the project—has taken steps to build personal rapport. Research teams should make a conscious effort not to be seen as some sort of clubby in-group; everyone involved in the research should adopt comparable and appropriate membership roles, a concept to be discussed below.

The Process of Collecting Information by Means of Naturalistic Observation: The Procedural Arc

Although we will have more to say in due course about procedures for recording and analyzing observational data, it is appropriate at this point to note that all observation-based inquiry tends to be carried out in a typical procedural arc (Spradley, 1980, pp. 33–34; Werner and Schoepfle, 1987, pp. 262–264).

The descriptive phase.

The process begins with **descriptive reporting**. This initial phase of the process relies on general questions that allow researchers to develop an overview of the site (e.g., the physical characteristics of both the place and the people). Descriptive observation may require researchers to adopt a child-like role, to assume that they need to record all perceptions without yet making assumptions about which ones are relevant. Descriptive observations should also be unencumbered by interpretation. For example, an observation note from the monastery study in the descriptive phase of the project might simply say, "One of the brothers read aloud from the Bible while the rest of the monks ate dinner," not "The monks are all interested in scripture study."

The focusing phase.

At the point when it becomes easier to sort out the irrelevant from the relevant, **"focused" observations** can begin; researchers observe factors of particular interest with greater intensity, although they never lose sight of how those factors fit into the larger context of the site as a whole. Focused observations often concentrate on well-defined types of activity or events (e.g., religious rituals, sporting events, political rallies) that lend themselves to the discovery of patterns or regularities in behavior, as opposed to unique or random occurrences. Repeated observations in the refectory (dining area) of the monastery might yield a note such as, "The monks are allowed to go back for second helpings, but almost never do so." The discernment of patterns should ideally lead to clearly stated research questions, which take the place of the more formalized hypotheses of quantitative inquiry. ("What social skills must novice monks learn in order to live in community? How do they go about assimilating such knowledge into their everyday behavior?")

The selective phase.

Such questions can only be addressed with **"selected" observations**, which allow the researcher to establish and clarify the relationships among elements in the site. Spradley characterizes the progression from descriptive to focused to selected observations as a kind of funnel, where researchers' attention is both narrowed and deepened as the research progresses. He cautions us, however, that "even as your observations become more focused, you will continue making general descriptive observations until the end of your field study" (1980, p. 33).

The saturation point.

The funnel ultimately tapers to a **saturation point**, which occurs when new findings consistently replicate material that has already been discovered and accounted for. It may be appropriate to suspend data collection when saturation is achieved and commence the process of analyzing the data. We will have more to say about analysis later on, but it should be kept in mind that because observations, like other kinds of qualitative data, are sometimes recorded in narrative rather than numerical form, there are particular challenges inherent in the process of retrieving and making sense of them. This is where the systematized nature of social research becomes particularly important: no matter how acute the observations may be, they are useless unless they are clearly recorded and readily available for retrieval and analysis.

How a Naturalistic Observer Takes Notes

For this reason, it is very important that observations be **recorded in a systematic fashion**. There is no universally accepted format for doing so: some researchers prefer highly structured check-lists, grids, tables, and so forth, while others choose free-form narratives. Some enter data directly into computer software programs, while others use more traditional means like notebooks or index cards. Group projects require that a standard method be adopted and used by all participants. Although these specific procedures will be dealt with in greater detail below, a few basic principles of note-taking may be suggested at this point:

- Every note should be headed by the date, place, and time of observation, regardless of the medium selected for recording.

- As many verbatim verbal exchanges as possible should be recorded (except in those rare situations in which only non-verbal behavior is the subject of study), as nothing conveys the sense of "being there" better than the actual words of participants.

- Pseudonyms or other codes should be used to identify participants in order to preserve anonymity and confidentiality. (See the section on ethics below for a discussion of why these cautions are in order.

- Events should be recorded in sequence so that upon repeated observations it will become clear which elements in the process are regular and patterned and which are random or optional.

- Basic notes should be free of inferences and interpretations, although some researchers like to keep personal journals (separate from their research notes) in which to record such speculations for future reference.

Evaluating Data Collected
by Means of Naturalistic Observation

Both the collection and analysis of observational data have been dogged by questions of **validity** and **reliability**. This hotly contested topic has been treated in great detail by Kirk and Miller (1986), but a few important points can be stressed here.

Validity.

"Validity" refers to the degree to which research findings somehow match up with reality. We all know that in real life, multiple eyewitness accounts of the same event can vary wildly—the famous "Rashomon effect"—such that even the criminal justice system is reluctant to rely on them exclusively. How, then, can we be sure that what researchers tell us about their observations is anything more than their take on the matter, no better or worse than anyone else's? We might rightly suspect personal bias in the accounts of people and activities derived from observational research. Researchers therefore like to "triangulate" their methods as much as possible—using several different sources of information (e.g., relying on interviews and/or archival materials to supplement observations) to converge on a comprehensive picture. They can also work in teams so that several different researchers are recording and analyzing observational data using standardized methods; in such projects, any idiosyncratic findings can be discarded and "reality" is held to be the point at which there is convergence among the observers.

As the use of video recording technology becomes more widespread, it becomes possible to preserve a visual record of an event and the people involved therewith, such that the intended audience can "see for themselves" that researchers have correctly reported on the scene. It should be kept in mind, however, that no recording system yet devised can also capture perceptions that come to us via the other four senses—perceptions that would inevitably make the experience of researchers who were on the scene different from that of audience members seeing only a visual record. Some qualitative researchers also speak of using "verisimilitude," a way of reporting findings that is so evocative and compelling that the reader believes the report to be "authentic" (Atkinson, 1990). This standard, however, is widely contested; after all, those researchers who happen to be poor prose stylists incapable of engaging the reader should not be assumed to have engaged in faulty observations that should be disregarded.

Reliability.

"Reliability" refers to the degree to which there is consistency in the research process; in the natural sciences, for example, the same experiment when repeated should yield substantially the same results every time, regardless of who is conducting the experiment. The degree of fit can be measured statistically. Outside the controlled experimental setting, however, qualitative inquiry is conducted by real people (with their own personality quirks as well as the categories—gender, race, class, age, and so forth—by which they may be socially defined) interacting in some way with other real people. It would be impossible to eliminate that personal variation, and a growing body of opinion holds that we should *not* eliminate it, as it is an essential part of the context we are studying. Even if a report is taken as valid for the reasons discussed above, how do we know that it is reliable enough to allow for generalization beyond the case at hand? It is certainly true that systematizing observations and repeating them with care—in imitation of the classic scientific method—over a period of time will help convince skeptics of the reliability of the findings. If the systematic observations are done under varying conditions (e.g., time of day, specific locale) and still yield the same findings, we can be reasonably confident that the procedures themselves are reliable in that they seem to be reasonably unaffected by extraneous factors. It should be noted, however, that increasing numbers of qualitative researchers would reject the notion that any factors that are part of the "natural" setting are in any way extraneous. They would also question whether we should try to emulate the scientific model at all; the carefully documented particular case can, under the right circumstances, be as valuable as the delineation of a proposition that seems to apply in a generic sense.

Observer Roles

The distinction made earlier between unobtrusive or non-reactive observations and observations based on researcher participation may lead to the conclusion that the types of observational research fall into a neatly dichotomized system. The situation is, however, both more complex and more interesting, as research is best understood as falling along a continuum defined by the roles assumed by the researcher. In the classic typology of researcher roles (Gold, 1958) there are four main points along the continuum. Observations can be conducted by researchers playing any of these roles, or even operating at the margins where the roles shade into each other. The adoption of a particular role sets limits on what the researcher can observe in the first place and on how he/she can analyze it later on.

Complete participants.

Complete participants are those whose observations reflect their status as thoroughly enculturated insiders to the setting under study. Complete participants certainly have the advantage of already knowing many things about the setting; on the other hand, they may also have a tendency to take many things for granted. They might also be compromised because pre-existing ties to other members of the group might make it difficult to provide an accurate rendering of what is occurring. There are, it should be noted, a number of researchers who take the position that such complete-immersion subjectivity, while far from the traditional scientific ideal, is valid on its own terms, in which case personal autobiography becomes a path toward an understanding of the larger social processes in which the individual is enmeshed. Social scientists in the "autoethnography" genre "not only observe the world around them, but also examine their internal perceptions and feelings about their place in the world" (Berger and Ellis, 2002, p. 156; see also Ellis and Bochner, 2000). For them, it is an explicit methodological choice to eschew traditional scientific detachment, and while their position is by no means the norm, it is becoming increasingly acceptable.

Participants-as-observers.

Insiders who are able to step back from time to time in order to record the scene in an objective manner (i.e., to see the scene independently of their autobiographical interest in it) become **participants-as-observers**, according to Gold. Such people are "indigenous" to the social setting under observation. Smith (2005, p. 96) refers to them as "native scientists" who "intend to contribute to change for the benefit of [their] communities, to ensure that science listens to, acknowledges, and benefits indigenous communities." The words "indigenous" and "native" tend to conjure up images of people from "exotic" locales, but it is possible to be a participant-as-observer in settings closer to home. For example, I was once commissioned to do a study of my own professional association, the Southern Anthropological Society, a group with which I had been affiliated for more than three decades (Angrosino, 1997). My oral history interviews with members were conducted in the context of a detailed, systematic observation of the group's annual meeting, in which I was also participating as a paper-presenter and member of the executive committee. I had been attending such meetings regularly ever since I was in graduate school, but this was the first time I made conscious, formal notes about what I observed.

Observers-as-participants.

   With a small, but very important, shift in nuance, we can move along the continuum to the **observers-as-participants**: outsiders who enter the study community explicitly for the purpose of conducting research. While they might stay in (or in proximity to) the community for an extended period and therefore come to be thought of as an everyday part of the scene, it is always clear that they come from "outside" and will ultimately go back once the research is concluded. This role is the one adopted by the pioneering cultural anthropologists of the early twentieth century and "participant observation" of this type has become widely popular among professionals in the many other disciplines who employ the ethnographic method. (See Hume and Mulcock, 2004 for a collection of reflective essays on the contemporary practice of participant observation.)

Complete members.

   Most contemporary researches seek some sort of "membership role" in this participant observation tradition. Those who adopt the **complete member** role seek to lose their outsider identification almost entirely and become totally identified with the community under study. In earlier generations, this shift was referred to rather pejoratively as "going native," the implication being that such researchers gave up their scientific credibility by becoming supposedly uncritical insiders. But, as noted above, because there is increasing tolerance for a more autobiographical approach to ethnography, the adoption of complete membership is no longer automatically stigmatized. Applied social scientists, for example, sometimes become advocates for the people they have studied, a commitment that extends long after the research per se has concluded. Gwynne (2003, p. 135) describes the anthropologist Rhoda Halperin as "an ardent defender of her study population, members of a working-class community." Halperin is said to identify "passionately" with the people of the neighborhood, "viewing them as representatives of oppressed working-class people everywhere who are trying to resist the powerful forces of urbanism and capitalism that are threatening to obliterate their culture." Moreover, she sees it as part of her ongoing role to "educate outside urban planners" about the needs and goals of the people of the community; note that she refers to the planners as outsiders, implying that she has come to see herself as an insider.

Active members.

The more typical choice, however, remains the role of the **active member** who, like the participant observer in the standard anthropological tradition, remains an engaged outsider. Some researchers, by contrast, seek the **peripheral member** role, involving proportionately less identification with the people under study. Peripheral membership may be advisable when the study community is engaged in behavior that is at best questionable and at worst illegal. Bourgois' (2002) study of urban drug dealers and Dalla's (2000) study of sex workers both benefited from the rapport developed by these intrepid researchers with respect to their research subjects; but it would clearly have been counterproductive for either of them to have become so active in their study communities that they themselves were subject to assault or arrest.

Evolving members.

Sometimes, the membership role preferred by a researcher turns out not to be one that is agreeable to members of the study community; when this occurs, the relationship is often modified in order to satisfy members' concepts of what is acceptable. For example, Behar (1993) wanted to tell the story of Esperanza, a poor Mexican Indian woman who had defined herself through her life's struggles. Behar was drawn to this woman, whom she first met while the latter was selling flowers on a street corner, because she felt that by understanding Esperanza, she might come to a better understanding of her own status as a Cuban immigrant in the U.S. who had always felt outside the social and academic systems in which she sought membership. Behar initially thought she could play the role of prestigious outsider to whom Esperanza would accord due deference, and who would automatically accede to participating in the research with no further questions asked. She was quite surprised when Esperanza reacted in a "haughty" manner and in other ways tacitly declined to play the part of the oppressed Third World woman. She did not even care to play the "exemplary feminist heroine" (1993, p. 270). Behar responded to Esperanza's challenge by questioning her own assumptions about the power relationship in ethnographic research, feeling herself to be directed by the more assertive woman she wished to study. Esperanza refused to fit into the category of "research subject", and so Behar had to redefine her role in Esperanza's world. Doing so ultimately meant that she became part of Esperanza's family network, which involved her becoming the godmother of Esperanza's daughter.

Complete observers.

Finally, there are **complete observers**, the outsiders who remain outsiders, whose aim of uncompromised objectivity is facilitated by their detachment from the people under study. In some cases, complete outsiders are not only unknown to the community as individuals; they are not even identified as researchers. The sort of observations that could be conducted without attracting notice in public space lend themselves to the adoption of this role. At one time in the not so distant past, this brand of non-reactive observation was considered the most appropriate way for social scientists to conduct research, as it most closely paralleled the kinds of observations natural scientists might conduct of experimental subjects in a laboratory. (See, e.g., Webb, Campbell, Schwartz, and Sechrest, 1966.) Nowadays, however, the complete observer role strikes some ethnographers as vaguely voyeuristic (particularly if it involves photography). Although it may actually be exempt from standard forms of research ethics review (see below), non-reactive research is predicated on the ability of observers to essentially hide in plain sight; concealing one's identity as a researcher can come uncomfortably close to deception. In any case, unobtrusive observation has by no means become the norm, particularly as qualitative social scientists have expressed a strong preference in recent years for admitting to a degree of subjectivity in their work; complete objectivity, even if possible to achieve, is now seen as a less desirable way of investigating the deeper meaning of a social setting.

For Discussion

1. Think about a piece of qualitative observational research that you might like to carry out. Start with a topic or theme that you want to learn about. You can begin with a theoretical interest (something you have already studied in other contexts) or with an interest derived from current events. Consider the site(s) at which you can most fruitfully pursue your inquiry. Keep in mind your own comfort level as well as the scholarly salience of the possible site(s). What, if anything, needs to be done in order to secure entrée into the site(s)?

2. Select a role for yourself as an observer and discuss the pros and cons of adopting such a posture. In what ways can you address the questions of validity and reliability in your project? Present your reflections to an appropriate group of peers and discuss the similarities and differences in the various approaches.Select any piece of empirical social research in your field that makes significant use of observational techniques. Explore the methods of the author(s). Evaluate the process for choosing the research site(s). Examine the choice(s) made about role; how did the choice of role affect the outcome of the study? Assess as best you can the validity and reliability of this study. Present your reflections to an appropriate group of peers and discuss the similarities and differences in the various approaches.

Chapter Two

Naturalistic Observation: An Overview of Some Influential Schools of Thought

Naturalistic Observation: An Overview of Some Influential Schools of Thought

One of the foundational techniques of social research, naturalistic observation is practiced in many different academic disciplines and professional fields. With regard to qualitative research in particular, there are certain schools of thought whose influence cross-cuts many of those disciplines and that have had a major impact on the way we understand the nature of observation, and the ways in which it might be applied to an understanding of human social behavior.

The Early Field Tradition, Historical Particularism, & Functionalism

The first approach to field-based research, popular around the turn of the twentieth century, involved social researchers joining scholars from other disciplines on large expeditions to remote parts of the world; while their colleagues studied the flora, fauna, and geological features of the region, the social scientists busied themselves with descriptive reports about the people of the area. Since such expeditions were usually mounted from ships anchored off-shore, there was not really much time to do a proper job of social research. At best, it was a matter of "quick forays into accessible villages and settlements" (Barrett, 1996, p. 73)—better than nothing, but not a firm basis for the development of a study of culture and society in the modern sense. It was not until the eve of World War I that there was recognition of the

desirability of having well trained researchers conducting extended fieldwork derived from their own sense of socially important topics, and not from whatever could be accomplished around the margins of other scientists' research. By that point, advocates of two parallel theoretical movements— **historical particularism** in the United States and **functionalism** in Britain— reached the conclusion that the study of social institutions and their - supporting culture could only be understood by the accumulation of empirical, descriptive data emerging from on-site observations of people and their activities. Both of these schools of thought consciously reversed the nineteenth century "grand theory" tradition (a **deductive** approach to inquiry that began with general theoretical propositions that could be used to generate testable hypotheses) by starting with ground-level observations and working up toward explanatory models (an **inductive** model of inquiry). (See McGee and Warms, 2004, pp. 128-215 for more details on these schools of social theory.)

Symbolic Interactionism

Another widely influential approach to the study of society and culture is **symbolic interactionism**, which emerged from sociology and social psychology in the 1920s. Interactionists share with the historical particularists the belief that society is not a relatively stable set of interlocking institutions, but rather a kind of shifting kaleidoscope. Unlike the historical particularists, however, they identify the pieces of the kaleidoscope not as "traits," but as individuals ("actors") whose actions, productions, and thoughts are shaped by interactions with other individuals rather than by academic abstractions like "the culture" or "the social structure." For interactionists, people are active agents and not interchangeable parts of a large system, passively acted upon by forces external to themselves.

Despite their philosophical differences with both the historical particularists and the functionalists, the interactionists readily agreed with the emphasis on first-hand fieldwork that had been developed in those schools. The purpose of field observation for the interactionists, however, was to uncover the meanings social actors attach to their actions. Some interactionists refer to their brand of observation as "sympathetic introspection," although others prefer to use the German word **verstehen**, which was coined by the influential German sociologist Max Weber. This research technique requires researchers to become subjectively "one" with their subjects, not neutral observers of them. The goal of interactionist field observation is to uncover the system of symbols that gives meaning to what people think and do.

Symbolic interactionists have extended their interest in the interactions among the actors in the settings they are studying to an analysis of the interactions that are part of the process of fieldwork itself. In other words, they have fostered an introspective analysis of the ways in which observers are linked to those whom they observe. The typologies of observer roles discussed in the previous section reflect this interactionist concern for the ways in which researchers are situated with respect to those they observe. (See Herman-Kinney and Verschaeve, 2003 for a more complete discussion of the interactionist approach to social research.)

Ethnomethodology

Ethnomethodology is a school of social research that emerged in the 1960s. Ethnomethodologists share with the symbolic interactionists the assumption that social life is constructed by members of a social group as they interact with each other. They are, however, not particularly concerned with the meanings attached to behaviors and material products (on the assumption that people often do not know on a conscious level why they are doing things, so that their explanations are not necessarily more valid than any other interpretation). They are more inclined to study the *how* of social construction, rather than the *why*. The ethnomethodological approach is based on the collection of large amounts of behavioral data (preferably with the aid of both audio and video recording) which are then broken down into minute pieces for analysis by means of detailed notational coding systems. This system requires a degree of objectivity, even neutrality, which is very different from the interactionist goal of sympathetic introspection. The ethnomethodological approach focuses observations on very precise events; it is typically fixed in location (as opposed to the approach of interactionists who would characteristically follow their "actors" wherever they happened to go) and delimited by the immediate conditions under study (e.g., a particular conversation). (See Holstein and Gubrium, 1994 for further information about the ethnomethodological approach.)

For Discussion

1. Return to the research project you proposed in the previous section.
   Consider how the adoption of each of the traditions discussed in
   this section might differentially affect the way you conduct that research.
   Present your reflections to an appropriate group of peers, taking note
   of differences and similarities in your conclusions.

2. Return to the research you read about in response to the question in the
   previous section. To which of the traditions discussed in this section would
   you assign that study? How does it illustrate the principles presented
   above? In what ways does it diverge from those general principles?
   If you think your study does not clearly fit any of the types,
   how would you characterize its approach to inquiry?

Chapter Three

The Varieties of
Naturalistic Observation

The Varieties of Naturalistic Observation

There are three broad categories of observational research: the **unobtrusive** (non-reactive), the **reactive**, and the **participatory**.

Unobtrusive Observation

The basic premise of all forms of non-reactive research is that the people under study do not know that they are being studied. There are several types of unobtrusive observation that have been prominent in social research, representing different degrees of concealment by researchers and different modes of researcher interaction with their subjects.

Disguised observations.

Disguised observations require researchers to become part of the population being studied, but without letting the subjects know that they are conducting research. Disguised observers must be able to blend into the study population so thoroughly that they cannot be readily spotted as outsiders who are present for purposes other than simply doing whatever it is that everyone else is doing. The seminal research using disguised observation was Hall's (1966) study of "proxemic" behavior—the ways in which people in public places use body language and the arrangement of physical space to convey meaning beyond the spoken word.

Although there have been some recent studies conducted using disguised observation (e.g., Cahill, 2004), this sort of research is now considered to fall too close to the border of unethical behavior and is rarely used. The study that probably served as the alarm indicating the dangers of disguised observation was that of Humphreys (1975), who observed men using a public restroom as a place in which to engage in covert homosexual activity. Humphreys made himself an acceptable part of the scene by offering himself to the regulars as a "watch queen," whose role (a recognized part of the social structure of the homosexual community in that still largely closeted era) was to let the others know if someone not a part of their culture was entering the restroom. In this role, Humphreys was performing a valuable service to the members of his study population who were therefore not inclined to be too inquisitive about any other motives that might account for his frequent presence.

Regardless of one's personal view on homosexuality, most people would probably agree that the men Humphreys studied constituted a "vulnerable population" since some of the acts he observed them committing were illegal and could have led to their arrest had his data been subpoenaed. Even without the threat of legal action, many of the men would probably have suffered greatly had they been unwittingly "outed." The ethical standards of our own time would suggest that the anonymity and confidentiality of the people Humphreys was observing were at significant risk.

The reaction to the Humphreys controversy has varied widely. (See Bernard, 1988:302-303 for a summary of responses.) A few researchers have defended the method in general (although not necessarily the way Humphreys carried it out) by pointing out that certain kinds of behaviors that are by definition covert can only be studied by covert means. They also claim that public places cannot be off-limits to social research, no matter what improper, embarrassing, or even illegal activities people choose to conduct in such settings. On the other hand, there are those who insist that some public spaces—restrooms most particularly—carry with them a culturally sanctioned sense of "assumed privacy." To some scholars, this principle means that all disguised observation should by definition be out of bounds, virtually excluding the use of binoculars, bugging devices, peepholes and so forth; they argue that all observation in public spaces ought to be conducted in ways that are themselves of a public nature. Proponents of eschewing disguised observation altogether also make the case that since we can never foresee the potential harm that might come from research conducted without due attention to the principles of informed consent (see below), it must always be considered unethical. But the compromise position, as articulated by Bernard (1988, p.303, emphasis in original) seems to be the one agreeable to most: "The decision to use deception is up to you, provided that the *risks of detection are your own risks and no one else's*. If detection risks harm to others, then don't even consider disguised ... observation."

Naturalistic field experiments.

As stated at the outset, qualitative research does not typically operate by the principles of experimentation that characterize the biomedical sciences. There is, however, one specialized category of observational research, the **naturalistic field experiment**, which has been employed by a handful of researchers. A naturalistic field experiment is a situation that is created or manipulated by researchers in order to result in behavior that can be observed and analyzed. This technique is best employed when researchers want to know which behaviors are typical of certain situations; it is less effective when it comes to figuring out why people behave in certain ways. One of the frequently cited pioneers of the naturalistic field experiment approach was the social psychologist Milgram (see, e.g., Milgram, 1963). Like disguised observation, however, the naturalistic field experiment has been out of favor for several decades, because it seems overly manipulative.

Indirect observations.

Given the possible ethical conflicts inherent in covertly observing people as they are in the act of doing something, some researchers have turned to the observation of the effects left behind by those activities. Hence, such studies are called **behavior trace studies**. There is a serious question as to whether one can truly observe inanimate things in the same way one can observe people and active behavior; the indirect observation of effects left behind is perhaps more akin to the humanistic study of texts than to other forms of social/behavioral research discussed here. But it can certainly contribute to our understanding of human behavior. Researchers have, for example, found graffiti in public restrooms to be a rich source of information about cultural values (Sechrest and Flores, 1969). A study of cars in an urban junkyard revealed information about the average use-life of American vehicles, which appears not to be dependent on the initial cost of the vehicle (Gould and Potter, 1984). An analysis of the wear pattern on the floor tiles in a public museum demonstrated which exhibits were the most popular with visitors (Webb et al., 1966, p. 37). All of these studies are examples of the use of "behavior traces"—the artifacts left behind in the wake of human activities—to conduct an indirect study of those behaviors.

The most frequently cited example of a trace study is the exercise in "**garbology**" begun by Rathje and associates (1984). In addition to being a staple of the academic literature on social research, it has also captured the attention of the popular media and has long been used as a touchstone for "quirky" but interesting research. An archaeologist by training, Rathje was particularly interested in patterns of consumer behavior. To that end, he undertook the analysis of garbage from a representative sample of households in several American municipalities. So as not to tempt people to throw out only stuff that makes them look good, no one was informed that their garbage would be gone through, sorted, and analyzed. According to local laws in the study community, trash placed at the curb for pick-up is no longer considered to be private property. The researchers could not, however, examine anything that had been thrown into a kitchen disposal, set aside for recycling, or consigned to a back-yard compost heap. In order to preserve anonymity, any material that could be used to distinguish one household's set of garbage from another (e.g., bills, photos) was immediately discarded. One of the most striking findings of this project was that whenever people change their food consumption habits, there is an increase in food waste, at least in the short run; it has been suggested that when people are unfamiliar with a food product, they waste more of it experimenting with ways to prepare it. The garbologists also conducted a cross-cultural analysis by comparing Mexican American and Anglo households. They found that the former used a relatively limited set of foodstuffs with which they were already very familiar; the latter tended to include more variety in their food purchases. As a result, the Mexican American households had far less waste than their Anglo counterparts.

Trace studies can yield data that are amenable to standardization and quantification. Comparisons across time and across populations are possible. A good case could also be made that these studies are more accurate than observations of actual behavior, particularly when the study population is unaware that the "traces" they have left behind in public places are subject to analysis. Figuring out what people eat is presumably easier when one analyzes the remains of their meals than when one asks a direct question, as people's responses may vary due to faulty or selective memory. (See Freeman, Romney, and Freeman, 1987 for a more complete discussion of these points.)

Reactive Observation

Reactive observation (or "direct" or "structured" observation) occupies a middle ground between unobtrusive observation (whose practitioners attempt to adopt the "complete observer" role vis-à-vis their study populations) and participant observation (whose practitioners attempt to adopt a membership role of one sort of another in their study populations). What differentiates reactive observation from unobtrusive observation is that the people being observed know that their behavior is being recorded. These two forms of research are similar, however, in that they are best suited to the description of what people do, rather than to the analysis of why they do it, or what their behavior means to them. This quality links reactive observation as a method to the theory of behaviorism that displaced the meaning-centered psychoanalytic school of personality in the 1950s. What differentiates direct observation from participant observation is that the researcher is known to the study population strictly as a researcher—he or she makes no attempt to "hang out" or interact with the members of the group except for the explicit purposes of the research project. It is a style of research that was initially developed by **ethologists**, scientists who study the behavior of animals (Lehner, 1979), and as such it has been approached gingerly by scholars of human behavior. It is not, as Bernard (1988, p. 287) notes, "a 'friendly' technique." There are two varieties of reactive observation that have nonetheless had some impact on the study of human groups.

Continuous monitoring.

Researchers who employ the technique of **continuous monitoring** observe their subjects for a designated period of time, recording their behavior in minute detail throughout that period. This approach has found favor in the field of business and management (where it often takes the form of time-and-motion studies of workers) (Niebel, 1982; see also Borman, Puccia, McNulty, and Goddard, 2002; Sproull, 1981). It has also been employed by clinical psychologists studying behavioral disorders (Fassnacht, 1982), by educational researchers studying teacher-pupil interactions (Guilmet, 1979), and by criminologists studying police-civilian interactions (Sykes and Brent, 1983). One very notable continuous monitoring study was conducted by the anthropologist Richard Lee, who analyzed the way !Kung Bushmen in southern Africa manage to find subsistence in their resource-poor desert environment. He followed a band as the men hunted game and the women gathered plants. Much to his surprise, the !Kung were able to meet their basic food requirements by working less than two and a half hours per day per food producer; as such, they had considerably more leisure time than anyone would have predicted—

the common assumption prior to that study being that "primitive" people had to spend almost all their time and energy just to meet basic subsistence (Lee and DeVore, 1968).

Continuous monitoring studies are very often enhanced by video recording, which allows for the intensive analysis of micro-details of behavior. Video recording in this tradition goes back at least to the 1930s when Margaret Mead and Gregory Bateson shot extensive footage of Balinese dances and associated trance behavior (Belo, 1960). It is important to note that in all studies that have followed in this tradition, the camera is not hidden; its presence is obvious to the participants, who agree to be recorded and who, in some cases, are allowed to have the final say about the disposition of the footage. By general consensus, there is some self-consciousness at the outset of such projects, as the subjects are inclined to "play to the camera." But after a while the camera seems to become part of the ordinary scene and ceases to be a distraction (Albrecht, 1985; see also Kendon, 1979, cited in Bernard, 1988, p. 278).

Continuous monitoring has been attractive to those studying behavior that they cannot really participate in, such as the activities of drug users (Price, 2002). It has been particularly useful as a data collection technique for those studying the behavior of children. Interviews are tricky to conduct with children, who often cannot fill out survey questionnaires, and it is difficult to be a "participant observer" in the world of children when one is an adult. The most extensive, influential, and widely cited continuous monitoring project dealing with children is the Six Cultures Study directed by John and Beatrice Whiting (1975). Teams of researchers were assigned to field sites in Okinawa, Kenya, Mexico, the Philippines, India, and the United States (specifically a town in New England) where they made a total of 3,000 five-minute continuously monitored observations on equal numbers of boys and girls. The investigators all used the same methods to observe and record; they wrote out in narrative form everything they saw the children doing during the observation periods and also noted aspects of the physical and social environment in which the children's behavior was occurring. The data were sent to a separate team of researchers (who had not been in the field) to sort into categories. Because the resulting database is so large, statistically valid associations have been ascertained from the analytical process. For example, a culture's core values seem to be assimilated by children by the age of six; it is obvious that the values themselves will vary from one cultural setting to another, but it is striking that the process of transmitting those values seems to occur in accordance with a developmental time-line that transcends culture.

Spot sampling.

As distinct from continuous monitoring, **spot sampling** (sometimes referred to as "**time allocation study**") is predicated on researchers appearing at randomly selected places, at randomly selected times; their task is then to record what people are doing. Spot samplers assume that if a sufficiently large number of representative acts is recorded, then the percentage of times people are seen doing certain things approximates the percentage of time they spend on those activities (even when they are not being observed). It is the randomness of the observations that makes the results compelling when clear patterns emerge over the course of repeated recordings. Spot sampling has generally been used to study the same topics (especially with regard to work, the division of labor, and the allocation of resources) that have been the subjects of continuous monitoring projects; its proponents claim that its randomization procedures allow for the capture of a greater degree of spontaneous and "natural" behavior. (See, e.g., Erasmus, 1955; Johnson, 1975; Oboler, 1985; Scaglion, 1986.)

Participant Observation

When a qualitative research project turns from descriptions of human behavior to attempts to sort out meaning and motive, there is really no substitute for observational data collection based on some sort of membership role in the community under study. When researchers interact with the people they study in ways that go beyond the simple researcher-and-subject model of reactive observation, and when they carry out their observations from the perspective of an insider to the group, they are said to be practicing **participant observation**. There are several key reasons for choosing a participant role as the foundation for research:

- Being something of an insider gives a researcher entrée into settings and situations (e.g., intimate domestic life) that would be closed to the stranger.

- Participant observers are less apt to be sources of distraction than reactive observers; they become so much a part of the everyday scene that people do not bother to consciously modify their behaviors to accommodate their presence.

- Participant observation is a very effective platform for conducting further research. For example, in order to conduct meaningful interviews, or construct survey instruments that people in the community will be likely to respond to, it is very helpful to have something of an insider's perspective. Data collection instruments composed in researchers' offices or labs may have the benefit of objectivity, but they are not very likely to

be in tune with normative expectations, values, and attitudes of the study community and so may easily be ignored or answered in a less than thoughtful manner.

• While it remains important to ask people what they think is going on in a behavioral setting under study, it is also helpful when researchers themselves come to be familiar enough with the setting to have some ideas of their own about what it means and why it is important.

Being a participant observer probably strikes many novices as being more fun than other forms of research. It certainly has a glamorous cachet attached to it—the romance of the old-time anthropologist going off to live in remote and exotic locales for extended periods of time—that makes the relatively antiseptic practices of unobtrusive and reactive observers seem rather blah. But a research strategy should never be selected just because it seems to promise drama and excitement. All of the genres of research discussed in this section have legitimate roles to play, and each of them is particularly well suited to the study of certain social issues.

Moreover, being a participant observer is not without personal cost; adopting the role may require a degree of immersion in the study community that makes it difficult to simply go home or back to the office and tune it all out. The more one is involved in the life of a community other than one's own, the more one is prone to experience **culture shock**, the unsettling feeling that one is somehow adrift in a sea of unfamiliar people, activities, symbolic cues, and so forth. And the setting need not be wildly different in order to provoke such a response; most of us live in a zone of comfort that we very carefully construct around ourselves, such that even a relatively slight modification in routine or a reordering of what is expected can be distressing. The fact is that we are, in a sense, invading the privacy of those we have descended upon in order to study. It should not surprise us when they express curiosity about us and invade our private space in return—but even knowing that this is likely to happen does not always prevent us from feeling a bit of panic when it does come to pass. We need to be aware of these potential problems, but they need not be insurmountable barriers.

The bottom line is that participant observation requires a degree of self-awareness that goes beyond that which is advisable for practitioners of other forms of field research. Once we have a good sense of who we are— not only as researchers, but also as human beings—we are more likely to be able to be effective participant observers. (See Tierney, 2002 for a case study illustrating these issues.)

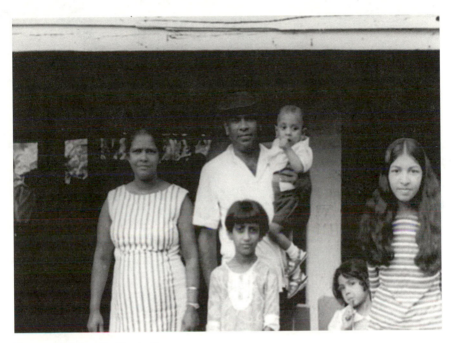

Figure 1: A Family Portrait

This and other photos were taken in the course of my research in Trinidad, which is discussed throughout the book. Use these photos to practice your observational skills. In this photo, what can you observe about the Trinidad Indian family? What questions do your observations suggest for further investigation?

There would, of course, be no point to participant observation if the emphasis were placed strictly on the "observation." It is a strategy for collecting data that relies on the ability of researchers to become involved on an everyday human level with the people they study. Indeed, most of the richest information in participant observation comes from encounters that might seem more like ordinary conversations than formal, planned interviews. Researchers cannot, however, depend on such encounters to materialize out of thin air.

Perhaps the most important skill needed to conduct participant observation—and the factor that tends to make or break such a research project—is the ability to cultivate good informants, members of the community who act not only as introductory gatekeepers, as discussed earlier, but who also continue to introduce us to others and who point us in the direction of relevant sources of information. Like "subjects" and "collaborators," terms that will be considered in the section on ethics below, "informants" is a word with somewhat unpleasant connotations, but it is the term most common in the literature, so we will continue to use it here.

Informants may be "general" in that they can serve as contacts with many people and have knowledge about many aspects of life in the study community. They may also be "key informants" who have specialized knowledge about selected aspects of life in the community. It is one of the ironies of participant observation-based fieldwork that researchers often end up with a broader and deeper knowledge of the community as a whole than anyone who actually lives there, since they have tapped into the specialized insights of a number of different people.

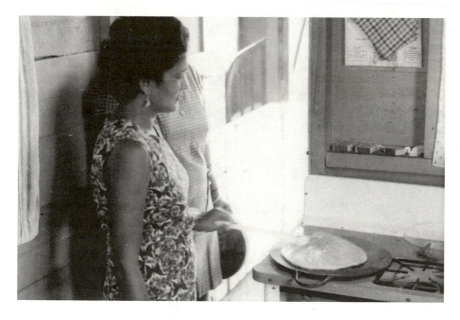

Figure 2: Women Cooking

What details of ordinary domestic life do you observe? In addition to the visual content of the photo, what sensory inputs might you expect in this scene (e.g., smell, touch, taste, hearing)?

Anthropologists, whose fieldwork has traditionally been of a long-term nature, have historically developed very close personal as well as working relationships with their informants. The special relationship between anthropological participant observers and their informants has been celebrated in studies both old (Casagrande, 1960) and new (Grindal and Salamone, 2006). As Bernard (1988) has commented, good fieldwork is dependent on finding—and keeping—trustworthy informants who are "observant, reflective, and articulate" (p.179).

For Discussion

1. Return to the research project you proposed earlier. In your initial formulation you chose a role for yourself as an observer. At this point, vary your proposal and discuss the pros and cons of adopting the various positions discussed in greater detail in this chapter. Present your reflections to an appropriate group of peers, taking note of differences and similarities in your conclusions.

2. Return to the research you read about earlier. In your initial discussion you considered the role selected by the author. Now discuss the ways in which the research might have been reformulated had the author used the various observation techniques discussed in this chapter.

Chapter Four

Naturalistic Observation:
Procedures and Practicalities

Naturalistic Observation: Procedures and Practicalities

As noted earlier, the quality that distinguishes observation as a tool of research from observation as a casual, everyday activity is its systematic nature. In this chapter, we will consider the procedures by which observation is systematized so as to enhance the quality of research, as well as some of the mechanical aids to the collection and analysis of field materials.

Procedures

Triangulation.

Perhaps the most important tool for systematizing observational research is **triangulation**, a concept introduced earlier in the discussion of validity and reliability. Triangulation is the use of multiple data sources in an attempt to test the quality of information.

For example, in my Trinidad study, I used a mix of observational techniques in order to come up with what I hoped was a rounded, holistic portrait of life in an Indian community in the midst of a major cultural transition. My main method was participant observation. I boarded with an Indian family for more than thirteen months and was accepted as a member of their social circle. I attended gatherings of the extended family, religious rituals, weddings, and funerals as part of that circle. I also had access to the workplaces (both at the sugar mill and the oil refinery) where members of the extended family were employed. Given the strong emphasis placed on the family as a social institution in the Indian community, I could not have hoped for entrée into many of these settings without having first been accepted as a kind of outlying relative. My relationship with the family was reciprocal, although in the long run I suspect that what they gave me—essentially the wherewithal to complete my research, write my dissertation, and get my doctorate—outweighed whatever I was able to give them in return. Nonetheless, I did give them money for my room and meals. On a less tangible level, I served as the godfather for one of the young children, and through that important ritual connection I have remained connected to the network for more than three decades.

My participant observation was supplemented by a considerable amount of archival research, particularly records left by the old colonial administration dealing with the importation of Indian labor during the period of the indenture. From those records I was able to ascertain the percentage of people whose ancestors had worked on the estate from which the contemporary village had grown, as compared with those who had moved to the village more recently. I was able to verify a perhaps obvious intuitive hunch— that the more remote the village, the higher the percentage of people whose families had "always" been in residence. The village where I lived, situated physically between the old mill and the new refinery, had a relatively high percentage of "newcomers." There were also important sources of information stashed away in the private holdings of a local doctor who had inherited the papers of a missionary who had worked among the laborers on the old estate.

Another kind of observation involved spot sampling at both the mill and the refinery. In light of my lack of qualifications to do the actual work required at those sites, I could not be a full participant observer. But given the family connections, I was able to stop by at random intervals of my own choosing; observations conducted in the course of such visits were sufficient to allow me to distinguish between random behavior and that which was part of the regular routine of life in those settings.

In a similar fashion, the deinstitutionalization study involved intensive participant observation; I situated myself first as a classroom volunteer in a community program serving deinstitutionalized adults who had been diagnosed with both mental retardation and chronic mental illness. The majority of the clients in the program had been in trouble with the law and had been ordered to the agency by the courts in lieu of prison. They were therefore people triply stigmatized, and I could not have gained entrée in the first place—let alone developed rapport and a sense of trust—had I simply endeavored to "hang out" as a non-reactive observer.

Because I had access to the clients' rooms, I was able to study the "traces" of their behavior in the form of the artifacts they had chosen as decoration. Since the program's administrators did not restrict the clients in their choice of décor, I found the posters, photos, and other collectibles to be a most informative mirror of the men's personalities, as well as their values and aspirations. Studying their highly diversified "traces" in their chosen decorations helped me understand that, popular stereotypes aside, people with mental disabilities are manifestly not "all alike."

I ultimately was asked to serve on the agency's board of directors, in which capacity I had access to the minutes of board meetings going back to the foundation of the program. By analyzing those archives, I was able to trace in detail the development of the public policy of deinstitutionalization in our state, as well as the specific response of one group of concerned community activists to that policy.

These examples demonstrate the value of employing multiple sources of information. Of course, in both cases there were other kinds of ethnographic data collection involved (including interviews of various kinds); but just considering observational techniques, we can see the ways in which different perspectives fill in a larger picture. It is not that any one of those techniques by itself would have been "wrong"; but certainly using them in combination to reinforce hunches, to weed out non-standard behaviors, and to validate perceptions about what was meaningful to people, certainly raised the confidence one could have in any conclusions drawn from those observations.

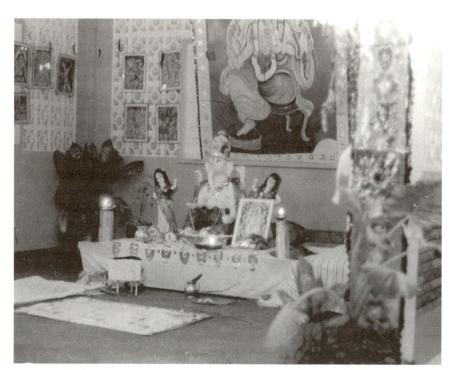

Figure 3: A Ritual.

*A puja is a Hindu devotional service; it can be either open to the public or celebrated in the privacy of a home. This picture depicts an altar prepared in honor of Ganesh, the elephant-headed god of wisdom and good fortune. Do you think this is a public or a private **puja**? What do the arrangements of the altar suggest about the nature of Hindu worship in Trinidad? Describe in detail what you see in this photo. What do you think you would be likely to smell, hear, touch, and taste, were you there in person? What questions would you like to ask a participant in this ritual?*

Pattern-finding.

Once a set of observations conducted via a reasonable variety of techniques has yielded a set of data, it is necessary for researchers to analyze those data. Analysis may be **descriptive** (concerned with breaking the data into its component parts to see if there are any discernable regularities, patterns, or themes) or **theoretical** (concerned with explaining why those perceived regularities exist). As Fetterman (1998, p. 96) notes, researchers "see patterns of thought and action repeat in various situations and with various players"; the search for patterns is therefore an important test of the **reliability** of the research, just as triangulation is a good test of validity. Finding patterns in data is a process not unlike creating a detailed index for a book.

Traditionally, patterns were discerned by manual means. Researchers would begin with a preliminary model, consisting of categories presumed to represent important features of the setting under study. This model might be derived from the available scholarly literature, although it would not likely remain within that framework; after all, there would be little point in collecting new data only to squeeze it into a categorization scheme devised for data collected earlier. In any case, it was important not to begin with too many categories; if there were many themes, then every incident could conceivably fall into its own category, making patterns impossible to discern. By the same token, having too few categories might mean that statements would be conflated, and behaviors that were actually distinct from one another would be treated as if they belonged to the same category. Written notes would then be sorted into those categories, but more than likely there would be things that either did not fit at all, or fit in several different places. This realization would lead to a revision of the model, the collapsing of some categories, and/or the creation of new ones. This process could go through several iterations before a satisfactory match between the model and the observed reality could be asserted.

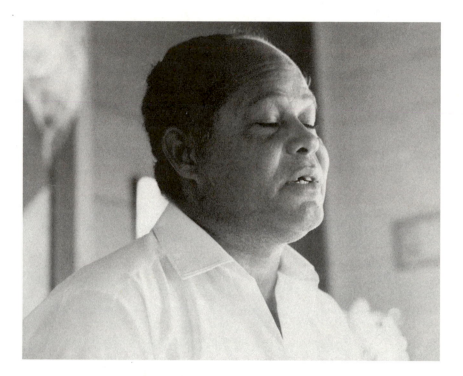

Figure 4: Man Addressing a Meeting of the Village Council

What emotions do you observe on the face of this man? What specific details about him stand out in your mind? Do you think he is a member of the council or simply a concerned citizen expressing his views before the council? What would you like to ask him if you had the opportunity to conduct an interview with him?

Database management programs.

Nowadays, this process may be streamlined by the use of database management programs specifically designed to handle the sort of narrative data typically collected by qualitative researchers. It should be noted, however, that such programs will only facilitate the matching of notes to categories and the highlighting of patterns within those matches; they cannot initiate the formulation of a working model or create the preliminary categories—that much is still left to the informed imagination of researchers. Researchers are also still responsible for deciding how to code their data—deciding, in effect, how to identify the "chunks" of data that can be sorted into one category or another. The main advantage of using a software program is that data, once entered, can be re-sorted as many times as necessary, with considerably less effort than would be required were manual means to be employed. Moreover, a software program operates via careful (virtually line-by-line) scanning of the data that have been input; in manual reading, it is possible to skim, and thus lose, potentially important pieces of information.

Most researchers nowadays are familiar with the basic computer functions entailed in **word processing** programs. Such programs do not merely facilitate the writing of the final report; they also allow for the creation of text-based files, and to find, move, reproduce, and retrieve sections of those texts. Word processing is also useful for transcribing and keeping track of field notes, and for coding text for purposes of indexing and retrieval. Another, perhaps less familiar, form of software is the **text retrieving** program, which locates each occurrence of a specified word or phrase, and which identifies combinations of such items in multiple files. **Textbase managers** have an additional capacity for organizing textual data. **Code-and-retrieve programs** assist researchers in dividing text into manageable sections, which can then be sorted. **Code-based theory builders** additionally permit the development of theoretical connections between and among coded concepts, resulting in relatively high-order classifications and connections. **Conceptual network builders** allow researchers to design graphic networks in which variables are displayed as "nodes" that are linked to one another using symbols to denote different kinds of relationships. Given the rapidity with which technology is changing in this area, I have avoided giving specific examples of these different genres of software; the reader is well advised to consult up-to-date websites containing the most recent information about specific programs.

Real and ideal behavior patterns.

Whether patterns are discerned manually or with the assistance of software, we can conclude that a meaningful pattern is *either* one that is shared by members of the group as manifested in their observed behavior, *or* one that is believed to be desirable, legitimate, or proper by members of the group, even if they do not always behave in accordance with that belief. We can therefore speak of patterns that are either **real** or **ideal**. Both are important and will be exhibited in each setting under study. Just because people do not always live up to their ideals does not mean they are duplicitous, just that everyday circumstances often militate against our acting out our highest ideals. Behaving in a less-than-ideal fashion does not mean that the ideals are meaningless, as they still are powerful shapers of our larger world view. In general, public statements and/or actions are more likely to reflect the ideal behavior of the group than are those expressed in private. Statements and activities that occur spontaneously or that are volunteered by people without prompting by a researcher are more likely to be elements in a shared pattern than are those that are expressed *only* in the context of a "naturalistic experiment" on the part of the researcher. (For this reason, naturalistic experiments are best conducted as part of a process of triangulation with other observational techniques, in order to verify the social and cultural salience of the behavioral pattern.)

Emics and etics in the analysis of behavior patterns.

When we conduct observations of any kind, and detect patterns in the behaviors of the people we are studying, we must always keep in mind that what might appear meaningful to us might not be so important to them—and vice versa. Social scientists sometimes refer to these two ways of looking at meaning in perceived patterns in terms derived from the study of languages. In linguistic analysis, phon*emics* is the study of sounds that convey meaning to native speakers of a language, while phon*etics* is the study of sounds that can be converted into an international code system that allows for the comparative study of meanings. So in the context of social research, an emic perspective is one that seeks patterns, themes, and regularities as they are understood by the people themselves, while an etic perspective is one that is applied by

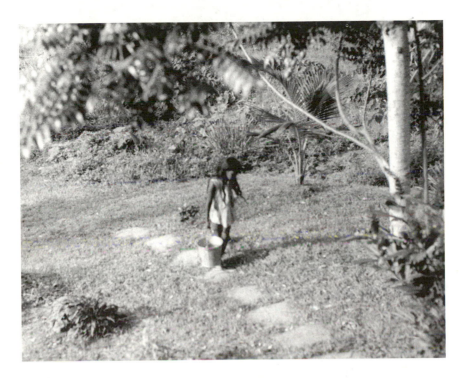

Figure 5: A child.

What do you think this child is doing? What is the physical setting in which she is carrying out her task? In addition to what you can see, what other sensory inputs do you think you would be aware of were you observing her in person? Does this image prompt you to want to know more? If so, what? How would you go about getting answers to your questions?

researchers (who will have at least read about, if not actually conducted first-hand observations in other communities) interested in seeing how what goes on locally compares to things happening elsewhere.

For example, in my monastic study, I observed a pattern of deference to the abbot. The monks would have interpreted this behavior as a response to the solemn vow of obedience they had taken; vowing obedience is a way of "dying to self" so as to make oneself more open to a relationship with God. While not discounting that emic explanation, I could also see that on an etic level, deference to some commonly recognized authority in many communities works to assure an orderly division of labor and provides a symbol of social cohesion.

In my Trinidad study, I was able to draw upon a large body of literature dealing with the system of indenture that the British used during the nineteenth century to transport Indian laborers to the far corners of the empire. From that literature, I was able to identify a number of themes that authors had used to categorize the history and current social situation of overseas Indian communities that had grown up in the wake of the indenture: the loss of caste; changes in family structure; the role of traditional religions; economic opportunities in the post-indenture period; political relations between Indians and others in the post-colonial society; secondary migration (i.e., second or third generation Indians leaving the place of indenture for the U.K., the U.S., or Canada). I began by organizing my notes according to these themes, but quickly realized that the first of them was inoperative. Except for Brahmins (the ritual specialists), most of the Indians in Trinidad were completely unaware of their traditional caste affiliations, and it was a matter of no importance to them. Even though many of them insisted that Indian culture in Trinidad was just the same as Indian culture in India, they were unconcerned with the whole matter of caste, one of the pillars of the traditional social order in their homeland. So other than affirming that there had indeed been a "loss of caste," my notes told me nothing more about this phenomenon. On the other hand, alcoholism emerged as a very important issue. The traditional Indian religions (Hinduism and Islam) are both strongly opposed to alcohol consumption, and yet even the most cursory observations in Trinidad demonstrated that a real drinking problem existed. Notes on observations of drinking behavior (and behavior at meetings of Alcoholics Anonymous (A.A.), where Indians gathered to discuss their problem) were scattered throughout my files. By separating them into their own category, it became possible to compare and contrast alcoholism against such predisposing factors as religion, family, economic and political relationships. The original categorization in this analysis was etic because it derived from the comparative literature on the world-wide indenture system. However, the later modification reflected an emic approach, responding as it did to what I had observed as actually important in that particular community.

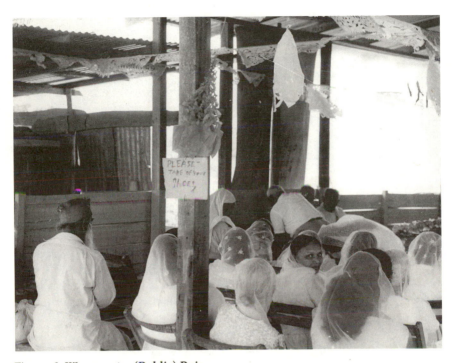

Figure 6: Women at a (Public) Puja

Can you discern any particular elements of Hindu public worship in Trinidad from observing this scene? What specific details stand out for you?

In the deinstitutionalization study, I used a preliminary model drawn from the literature with great caution, since so much of that literature derived from clinically based research and/or research conducted with the professional caretakers of people with mental disabilities. My observations revealed several important categories that might be said to represent broad areas of social concern: sexuality; finding and keeping a job; relations with family; relations with friends; relations with professionals; self-image. These emic categories were quite different from those emphasized in the literature, which were largely concerned with symptomatology and treatment modalities.

Presentation of Data

When data have been arranged into useful categories, it is possible to summarize them in text, tabular, or figure form (or some combination of these formats). There are several commonly used forms for the presentation of data.

The matrix.

In the context of social research, as opposed to the world of futuristic thrillers, a **matrix** refers to a table that compares two or more segments of a population in terms of one of the analytic categories. For example:

Hindu Indians	member of A.A.	not member of A.A.
Muslim Indians	member of A.A.	not member of A.A.

When the numbers of cases were filled in, it became clear in a way not apparent in the raw notes, that there were proportionately more Muslims in A.A. than the overall demographics might suggest. In the general population, Hindus accounted for 80% of Indians in Trinidad, and Muslims for 15% (the remainder were converts to Christianity). But Muslims made up 35% of the Indian A.A. membership. This presentation of data gave me ammunition to take my inquiry in a somewhat different direction: what accounted for the preference in one sub-community for alcohol rehabilitation? What other cultural distinctions could be discerned between Muslims and Hindus (despite the fact that the literature tended to treat them as all the same)?

The hierarchical tree.

A **tree** is a diagram showing different levels of abstraction in a theoretical analysis, with the most abstract categories at the top and the most specific at the bottom. For example, the process of deinstitutionalization could be described in the most general way in terms of two factors: political-economic forces that made community-based treatment seem like the most cost-efficient method, and humanitarian forces that made such treatment seem like the best way to insure respect for the dignity of persons with mental disabilities. A middle level reflected the kinds of relationships (with professional caregivers, family, friends, etc.) that would be encountered by deinstitutionalized people

regardless of whether the policy that put them in the community derived primarily from political-economic or humanitarian reasons, as such relationships would not have been relevant at all had they remained incarcerated. At the bottom were the specific observations I made of the people in the particular programs I was associated with.

Maps.

Maps are very useful visual aids in observational fieldwork, as it is often necessary to get the "lay of the land" in order to situate behavior in its proper context. Detailed published maps may be required if the scope of observations ranges over a very large area (e.g., an entire city, an island). It is possible nowadays to use geographic information systems (GIS) technology to augment information from conventional maps. GIS is essentially a computer system capable of capturing, storing, analyzing, and describing geographically referenced information. In other words, data are identified according to their location. GIS technology can help establish precise geographic coordinates for such locations as property boundaries, major structures, and natural features of the landscape that might have a bearing on the social situation under study. The technology helps a researcher relate information in a spatial context and to draw some conclusions about this relationship.

Most ethnographic projects, however, have a somewhat limited geographic focus and can make do with hand-made sketch maps. I have found the latter to be extremely useful in the ER study; although the ER is small in area, it is laid out in a maze-like pattern (a nurse once jokingly told me that it was deliberately designed that way to discourage people from trying to escape). I do not naturally have a keen sense of direction, my little map has been very helpful in getting around the area. An enlarged version of that same sketch map has been useful in helping to plot the location of the important human and mechanical resources that are needed to deliver ER services and to do a kind of time-and-motion study of how those people and machines get from one part of the ER to another. One may think of the published map as a guide to the "etics" of a community, while the hand-drawn sketch reflects the emic situation. In some cases, maps may be a useful tool for eliciting information, as when researchers ask informants to draw their own maps, or to comment on maps the researchers have drawn.

Counting and census-taking.

Two techniques often associated with ethnographic mapping are **counting** and **census-taking**. "Counting" in the context of observational research refers to "listing and enumerating types of people, material items, locations, or other things that are important in situating the event, location, or activity more accurately in the context of the community" (Schensul, Schensul, and LeCompte, 1999, p. 102). One does not need to be a high-powered statistician to see that descriptive observations are more compelling if we have an idea of how many people or things are involved. For example, writing, "There were a lot of people in attendance at the plenary session of the Southern Anthropological Society" is considerably less informative than writing, "Three hundred people, out of 350 registrants, attended the plenary session." There is certainly nothing wrong with impressionistic observations, but if it is possible to give some numerical shape to the data, then it is desirable to do so.

A census is a particular genre of enumeration: it is a list of every person, household unit, or anything else (e.g., livestock, farm equipment, bus stops, public restrooms) important in the study community. Large-scale census information is available in most places, but it is not always germane to local-level observations; in the latter case, it is often more helpful for researchers to enumerate the specific things they need (an emic view) rather than rely on categories established by government offices far away (an etic view). For example, once I had begun to see the salience of alcoholism in the Trinidad Indian community, I did a census of all the places where alcohol could be purchased (or otherwise made available) in a typical rural village. In addition to obviously marked "rum shops," there were grocery stores that sold liquor, as well as a number of private facilities that trafficked in "home brew." I was startled to find that in a village of not more than 1000 residents, there were no fewer than twenty outlets that regularly dispensed liquor.

Social indicators.

Among the most important things researchers can observe in the field are the material indicators of social behavior. Such indicators are the "behavior traces" discussed earlier, and it is sometimes useful to group data in terms of categories suggested by the social indicators at hand. Social indicators are particularly important when it comes to making observations about differentiations within a given community. Differential status can be marked by observing such characteristics as hair style, choice of clothing, type and amount of jewelry and body adornment, leisure activities, speech and language patterns, television or movie preferences, choice of car, and attributes of residences (the number of broken windows has famously been used to indicate "deteriorating" neighborhoods) (Schensul, Schensul, and LeCompte, 1999, p. 112). The deinstitutionalized men I worked with had a good emic social indicator of their own: those who bought their clothes at a store in the mall were considered to be "successful" in ways that those who shopped at the Salvation Army thrift store were not.

Flowcharts and organizational charts.

A flowchart is a kind of map, although it depicts the movement of people, products, or behaviors through a sequence of events. It is a particularly useful way of visualizing the steps of a routinized event (such as a religious ritual or an assembly line in a factory) so that it is possible to sort out the things that happen all the time from those things that might be random occurrences.

An organizational chart accomplishes much the same thing, except that it is a picture of a system rather than of a particular process within that larger system. Some formal groups, like businesses, schools, or hospitals, have very clearly defined (and often published or otherwise prominently posted) organizational charts; less formal groups may need to be charted by the researcher/observer in order to clarify a system that is recognized only implicitly by the participants themselves. The ER that I have been observing is part of a hospital that has a very detailed organizational flow chart that is published in all its promotional literature. The ER has its own chart, detailed to the point of depicting where each member of a trauma team is supposed to stand in orientation to the patient; a copy of that chart is posted prominently on the wall of each of the trauma bays. Some of my most fruitful observations have been to see when and how the actual practice deviates from the posted placements; I can then bring up perceived discrepancies when I interview members of the staff to discover which elements in the system are absolutely essential and cannot be varied from those that are optional, as well as from those that are never observed (i.e., that exist only in the minds of the planners who do not actually work in the ER).

Hypotheses/Propositions.

Unlike quantitative inquiry, which is based on the testing of formal hypotheses, qualitative research tends to be discursive in its narrative treatment of issues. Nevertheless, even qualitative data can be presented in such a way as to express the relationship between perceived variables. For example, I had observed that adult men with mental retardation who had active family ties were more apt to complete their community-based habilitation programs than those with weak or nonexistent ties. I certainly could not collect anything approaching a statistically representative sampling of all retarded men, even in my own town, let alone in general, and so testing a formal hypothesis was out of the question. I could, however, use this simple statement of apparent relationship as a way of organizing my data and understanding the life experiences of the men I was able to work with.

Metaphors.

Metaphors are literary devices, short-hand ways of expressing the quality of relationships. I like to think of them as poetic versions of the hypotheses/propositions of traditional scientific discourse. For example, in my Trinidad study, I had observed that Indians in the village lived in compounds—several houses in which several members of an extended family resided—behind a wall or fence. This architectural style seemed to be of a piece with the general Indian cultural preference for in-group exclusivity. One of my informants used the phrase, "Inside is life. Outside is death." He was referring specifically about his membership in A.A., but I also understood him to be reflecting the more general cultural attitude of Indians who saw the outside world as a political, economic, and cultural threat. For Indians, "inside" included family, religion, and jobs in the sugar industry, while "outside" included the political system of modern Trinidad, and jobs in the oil industry. As a result, even people who got jobs at the refinery because it was economically advantageous to do so felt a strong sense of cultural displacement. My informant's metaphorical division of the world proved to be a useful way to sort out my own data, and I ultimately used his phrase in the title of my dissertation.

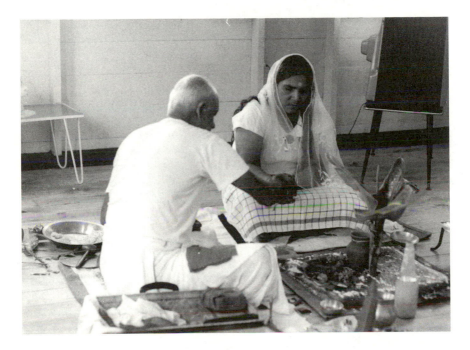

Figure 7: A Domestic Puja

How does the attitude of the woman in this photo differ from that of the women in the previous scene? How would you describe what is going on here? What do you think is the relationship between the man and the woman? In addition to what you can see, what other sensory input do you think you would be aware of were you attending the puja in person? What would you like to ask the participants? What are some other sources of information that might be useful to you in getting answers to your questions?

A somewhat cruder example of metaphor came from one of the deinstitutionalized men I studied, who lived in a room that I had observed to be noticeably messier than those of others in the program, even though he was not in other ways less socially functional than his colleagues. At one point he said to me, "My life is a toilet." He meant that he counted as a waste everything that he had ever done. One could take his remark at face value as nothing more than a cry of frustration or desperation. But it was also possible to use his home-made metaphor to unpack a lot of my observational data and to ask why it could be thought that life was a waste. Here was a man who had been fairly successful in his training program and who had already lined up a decent job in the community. But he (and many others, I discovered, even

those who did not express their feelings via the "traces" of a bedroom that looked like a junk pile) considered life a waste because he was not truly an adult: he was not trusted, he believed, to do many of the things adults do, including the very important matter of expressing his sexuality. As a result, he felt that everything he did was childish, and, hence, worthless.

Representation of Data

There is little point to collecting data and analyzing it so that patterns and themes emerge only to set it aside. There might be a certain satisfaction in doing research for its own sake, but most scholars want to engage in a conversation with other members of the scholarly community and also with interested members of the general public. When we convey data to an audience, we are engaged in the act of **representation**.

The scientific format.

It is often assumed that the only appropriate way to represent research data is in the form of the traditional scientific monograph, journal article, or conference presentation. The scientific format is designed to highlight the objectivity of the data, their analysis, and the findings. Its hallmark is a style devoid of the personality of the writer.

A scholarly report is headed by a **title** that should be a direct description of what the report is about. It should not be overly cute, although sometimes qualitative researchers are able to sneak in a colorful quote from someone in the study community to use in the title, as in my *Outside is Death*.

There follows a brief (100-200 words) **abstract**, which summarizes the basic research questions, the most important findings, and the methods used to collect the data designed to address those questions. There should be little or no explanatory or illustrative material in the abstract. In a book-length work, the abstract may be replaced by a **preface**, a longer statement that might involve a bit more detail.

The **introduction** to the text proper orients the reader/listener to the study. It includes a statement explaining (and, if necessary, justifying) the main research questions.

The first substantive section is the **review of literature**, a critical examination of the relevant published materials. Relevance, it should be noted, encompasses not only the substance of the research project, but also the theory and methods, which may have been developed for other topics, but which can be applied to the issue at hand. The review of literature is the place where the author's own theoretical framework and methodological orientation are explained and justified.

There is also a separate **methodological review** in which the procedures for data collection and analysis are presented. In the case of qualitative field research, this section may also include a description of the research setting, including both its physical characteristics and its demographic make-up.

The next section is the discussion of **findings and results**, in which the data collected in the study are linked first to the research questions posed in the introduction and subsequently to issues that emerged in the general review of literature.

A **concluding discussion** summarizes the main findings and suggests directions for future research. A study with an applied focus may also include **recommendations** for policy development or the implementation of service delivery programs.

At the back of the report are **references and appendices**, explanatory material supplemental to the main text. Depending on the preference of journal editors or book publishers, **notes** may be included in the text proper (as in this book), placed at the foot of a page, or grouped at the end of a chapter (or of an entire book). Notes are usually restricted to references; more substantial notes are usually avoided, as material important enough to mention at all should probably be in the text itself. There is a list of references cited at the end of the report; with the editor's permission there may also be a list of "other sources" not cited. References and citations follow strict scholarly form. As journals and book publishers have their own preferences for form,

it is advisable to have recourse to the authoritative source for such matters, *The Chicago Manual of Style* (2003). Appended materials might also include charts, tables, copies of original documents, and photos.

Subjective representations.

The scientific format was devised—and still works best for—the representation of research data collected through clinical or experimental means. When dealing with qualitative research, however, a degree of subjectivity necessarily comes into the picture; such research, after all, is produced out of the interaction of researchers and their subjects. The attempt at depersonalized objectivity is not always a comfortable way to represent qualitative field data. Ethnographers therefore may experiment with one or another form of alternative representation, or **reflexive narrative** of the lived experiences of the people they study and of their interactions with those people. These works fall into several main categories, sometimes referred to as "tales of the field" (Van Maanen, 1988; see also Sparkes, 2002). Alternative representations have the potential to reach audiences beyond the scholarly community (Richardson, 1990). As such, they may seem at first glance to be less rigorous than the kind of scientific reportage we are used to, but they can reach and move people, teaching them about the experiences of others in ways that are not possible in the scientific monograph—which, after all, is typically read only by other initiated scientists.

Realist tales.

Realist tales appear to hew closely to the scientific format, especially since the author remains conspicuously absent from the discussion. They are, however, characterized by extensive, closely edited quotations from the people who have been observed, with the intention of helping the reader "hear" the actual voices of the people whose experiences are being represented. Realist tales are therefore heavy on "local color" in ways that scientific monographs are not, even though such scene-setting is done in service to an objective account of the people and their setting. Realist tales have a long history, with the work of the anthropologist Bronislaw Malinowski as the classic example. According to Van Maanen (1988, p. 55), the author of a realist tale is required

to be a "sober, civil, legal, dry, serious, dedicated transcriber of the world studied"—although employing some so-called "swaying palms" scene-setting imagery is not off limits.

Confessional tales.

When the author steps out and becomes an actual character in the narrative, the result is a confessional tale. This genre explicitly recognizes the fact that the researcher is indeed part of the story—that the data would in fact not have existed were it not for the interaction of scholar and subjects. As such, the act of conducting participant observation, for example, is described along with the description of the community itself. Confessional tales rarely seem to stand alone; more often than not, there are confessional passages included in otherwise realist narratives. Manuals such as this book that elaborate on how to conduct ethnographic research are often full of confessional tales, as authors frequently use their own fieldwork experiences to illustrate basic principles. (See also Agar, 1980.) The term "confessional" may seem to connote the sharing of some shameful or even sinful secrets, but confessional tales are almost always upbeat in nature. They are often deployed to demonstrate how even mistakes made by a fieldworker resulted in the learning of important lessons. (See, for example, Lee, 1969.)

Perhaps the most elaborate and informative of confessional tales is the "thrice-told tale" of Wolf (1992). The book begins with a reprise of a fictional short story she wrote thirty years earlier when she accompanied her husband, an anthropologist, on his first field research in Taiwan. That story is followed by the field notes and journal entries she used when composing the story. Finally, there is a formal ethnographic article that Wolf (who in the meantime had become a professional anthropologist in her own right) originally published in *American Ethnologist*, a mainstream academic journal. Each section of the book includes Wolf's comments on what she remembers about the events as represented in each of the three written accounts, as well as what she thinks about them from the vantage point of three decades since the events took place. She notes an important change in her own understanding of her

professional role: "Where once I was satisfied to describe what I thought I saw and heard as accurately as possible, to the point of trying to resolve differences of opinion among my informants, I have come to realize the importance of retaining those 'contested meanings'" (p. 4).

Autoethnography.

In the confessional tale, the author is but one character out of many; in an **autoethnography**, also known as a "narrative of self," the author is the main character. Autoethnographers use their own personal experiences as the basis of analysis. Their tales are characterized by dramatic recall, strong metaphors, vivid characters, unusual phrasings (unusual in a scientific document, that is), and the holding back of interpretation so as to invite the audience to relive the emotions experienced by the author. The basic assumption in autoethnographic representation is that the researcher is a member of a cultural or social group, and that their personal experiences accurately mirror the experiences of the group as a whole. Indeed, since researchers are predisposed to be self-aware and analytical, the representations of their own experiences may be more acute than those of other members of the community. Ellis (1995), a sociologist by training, has written an extended narrative dealing with her experience of being the caretaker to a critically ill significant other and her reactions to his subsequent death. The details are particular to the case at hand, but Ellis' narrative style carefully links her specific concerns to general themes of life, death, and loss in our society.

Poetic representations.

While most representations of research data employ prose forms, it is also possible to use poetry as a means of expression. **Poetic representations** are forms of expression typical of the community under study, and they are offered as a way of giving the reader/listener a sense of how those people "see" the world around them. Poetic representations are not poems about researchers' own experiences or feelings; they are works that use the style and tone of expression typical of the community under study in order to describe experiences typical of that community. Richardson (1992), for example,

constructed a five-page poem about the life of an unmarried, southern, rural, poor, Christian woman. The poem was based on a thirty-six page interview transcript and used only the lady's own words; it was composed with careful attention to the voice, tone, rhythms, and diction of a person of this woman's time, place, and social station.

Ethnodrama.

Just as the poetic representation substitutes poetry for prose, ethnodrama uses theatrical scripts. Once again, however, the play is not about the researcher told in his or her own voice; rather, it is a way of using the community's own traditions of drama to convey information about life in that community. The resulting performance piece might include dance or mime as well as spoken dialogue, depending on local conventions. For example, Mienczakowski (1996) sought to enhance community understanding of mental health and addiction issues. To that end, he created two plays based on his ethnographic research in treatment facilities. The plays were performed with cast members drawn from the health professions as well as students of theater. Poehlman (2004) employed the technique of ethnodrama in the course of his study of HIV/AIDS prevention programs in Malawi, a nation in central Africa. After some time spent observing activities at rural health clinics, Poehlman devised a participatory strategy of involving local people in the research process. He collaborated with local health professionals in the planning and production of dramatic plays. The purpose of these productions was not didactic; the structure was not professionals teaching the local people about the disease but rather real-life situations depicting various social and cultural responses to the epidemic. The aim was to get the people talking about these scenarios and reflecting on positive and negative strategies for responding to relatives and friends who were at risk. Itinerant performers staging plays in the local language were already a common feature of the popular culture, so that these research-based dramas were not considered weird innovations by outsiders.

Fictional representations.

The fictional representation of social data does not mean that the data are made up. It refers, rather, to the use of the techniques of literary fiction (e.g., use of composite characters, setting characters in hypothetical events, attributing revelatory interior monologues to people when the researcher could not possibly have heard the original discourse, deploying flashbacks or flash forwards) to represent the experiences of the people under study. My own account of my research in community-based programs for deinstitutionalized adults (Angrosino, 1998b) is an example of the translation of ethnographic data into the form of short stories. In light of recent controversies about works labeled "non-fiction" that proved to have significant elements of the made-up, it is worth stressing that fictional tales in the research context (as opposed to the context of popular culture) are supposed to be clearly labeled as such. To repeat, they are fictional only in the sense of using literary tropes, not in the sense of inventing data.

Beyond the written word.

The filmed documentary has long been seen as a valid way to represent scientific data, often in conjunction with a published book (Heider, 1976). To be sure, filmmaking requires specialized skills that are not typically mastered by social researchers, although the advent of a new breed of **video technology** may ease the technological gap. Qualitative researchers may use the new **digital technology** to make expressive, fictional films (understanding "fiction" in the sense described in the previous section) in addition to objective documentaries. That same digital technology has made it possible not only to produce high quality images, but also to disseminate them in new and creative ways. It is possible to post both text and images on the internet, and while such **web-based representations** are still generally thought of as adjuncts to "real" publications, they are gaining in acceptance as more and more people have access to the web and seem to prefer it to other means of communication (Bird, 2003). A web posting is essentially an updated version of the visually-based museum exhibit of old.

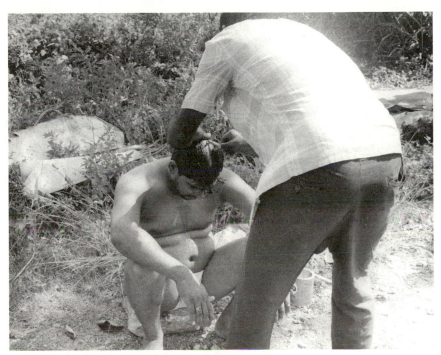

Figure 8: Man Preparing for His Father's Funeral

What does your observation of this scene tell you about a Hindu funeral in Trinidad? Does it suggest anything about family relationships? What do you think is the relationship between the two men shown in the photo? What else can you tell about the setting from observing this photo? What would you like to ask the participants? What other sources of information might help you understand what is going on?

Practicalities:
Mechanical Aids to Field Observation

Very few researchers have memories capable of storing and efficiently retrieving all the minute details that can be taken in during the course of observation-based fieldwork. We therefore all make use of mechanical aids to facilitate the process. Given the rapid evolution in technology, this section will deal only with major categories of mechanical aids, not with specific product recommendations. Readers are urged to do their own research to find out which current products best suit their needs within these general categories.

Notepads.

The most low-tech of all aids is, of course, the pad and pen/pencil. This tool may seem too obvious to merit any discussion, but its central importance to field research is such that it cannot be simply taken for granted. Hand-written and hand-drawn notes and sketches are often the first step in the long process of data recording and retrieval. Written notes and sketches made on the spot can later be translated into more formal (and legible) media, but since many researchers do not (or cannot) take their computers directly to the field site, all of us should learn to be careful when taking notes the old-fashioned way. At the risk of belaboring the obvious, it is necessary to go into the field with a sufficient amount of paper (a piece of advice from someone who, as a novice fieldworker, was once reduced to taking notes on the back of a candy bar wrapper) and something stiff against which to write in sometimes awkward situations. Pencils are good because they can be erased (so be sure to have a supply of clean erasers to accompany a good supply of pencils), although they have a tendency to smudge. Pencils that need frequent sharpening, or mechanical pencils needing frequent infusions of lead can be more trouble than they are worth. Pens are probably a better overall solution; creative types may want to bring along pens with variously colored ink in case they want to make some preliminary, color-coded analytic notations. If one is working in conditions where inclement weather may be part of the scene, it may be wise to invest in some of the rugged, weather-proof notebooks and waterproof pens favored by surveyors and field engineers. In any case, when using manual recording methods in the course of any kind of participant research, it is inadvisable to go around with one's nose buried in one's notebook; maintaining proper socially interactive eye contact and body language is probably more important than getting every last word down perfectly. For that reason, it is almost always advisable to go back over written notes as soon as possible; they typically have to be rewritten (or, more likely, typed into a computer file) so that they are legible and coherent.

Tape recorders.

Some of us are old enough to remember when **tape recorders** were the size of small pianos, used ever-so-fragile tape that had to be strung just-so between reels, and required bulky and obtrusive microphones in order to pick up any sound at all. (I recall a photo an older colleague once showed me of one of his informants, a frail elderly lady literally cowering in the shadow of a gigantic boom microphone. He used the photo as an ironic visual aid to his lecture on unobtrusive research methods.) Such machines were taken into the field only when absolutely necessary (e.g., when the project involved the collection of folk tales or music). Tape recorders have obviously gotten more compact and are relatively user-friendly as modern technology goes. As a result, they are now just about as common among fieldworkers as the notepad and pen. Their use in interview-based research is obvious, but even in situations requiring more observation than direct discourse, they are invaluable. They can pick up the ambient sound that forms part of the context of people's behavior. They can record the occasional comment that provides an important clue to the feelings of the participants. They can be used by fieldworkers who might feel more comfortable speaking their notes rather than writing them down (if, for example, they are concerned that someone might peek over their shoulder and read what they have written).

The **transcription of taped material** can be a very time-consuming process—and a rather expensive one if a researcher uses the services of a professional transcriptionist. These problems can be minimized when the tape is an adjunct to observations rather than the primary means of recording lengthy interview discourse. But it is still important for researchers to be sure to label their tapes clearly, record a "header" to each tape (that essentially repeats in verbal form the information on the written label), index them even if full transcriptions are not needed so that specific parts can be readily accessed when required, and store them in a manner that both preserves the confidentiality of anyone who may have been caught on tape and that is safe from the elements. As with simple paper and pen, researchers should be sure to carry a sufficient supply of tapes and batteries and perhaps even a back-up recorder just in case. They should also test their equipment before going out to the field; they should make sure not only that it is in proper working order, but that they know how to use it without fumbling when the crucial moment comes.

Some fieldworkers are now turning to **digital recorders**, which have the capacity to record and transfer information directly to a computer file, thus facilitating the organization, editing, and retrieval of notes. Some deluxe digital voice recorder (DVR) models include transcribers, which are essentially voice editing software programs. DVR's have considerably more recording capacity than old-fashioned reel or cassette tape.

Cameras.

Visual-based technology is changing at a rapid pace. The best state-of-the-art summary (as of this writing) is provided by Lally (2006).

Like tape recorders, **cameras** were once large, delicate, and expensive. Although field researchers have been using them since at least the 1930s, they did not become part of the standard equipment until they were reduced in both size and cost. Cameras play a vital role in all kinds of field research, but their contribution to observational research is especially noteworthy. The most important function of the camera in observational research is for the recording of physical behaviors and social interactions. Photographs are, in effect, "precise records of material reality" (Collier, 1967, p. 5). They are crucial in helping researchers reconstruct the settings so as to facilitate analysis of whatever happened in those settings. They can be used to illustrate major points in the final report. Cameras can also be shared with people in the community, who can be asked to take pictures of things important to them, thereby providing an emic glimpse into their world-view.

This latter function used to be handled by the now largely obsolete Polaroid camera, which allowed the researcher to take a picture and, within minutes, share it with the people involved in order to elicit their further commentary. Nowadays **digital photographic equipment** performs this same function by allowing people to see images even before they are printed on paper or onto computer files. Another recent innovation, the **disposable camera**, allows researchers to give these relatively inexpensive devices to people in a study community so that they can document their own lives; the results can then be shared and so become the basis for further discussion of behaviors, material objects, and other aspects of social life from an emic perspective.

As important as cameras are, their use cannot ever be taken for granted. There are still some communities in which the taking of pictures of people is considered socially inappropriate, and in certain political contexts, taking pictures even of buildings or apparently public places may be strictly off-limits. Even in communities where photography is generally appreciated and welcomed, there may be individuals who for any number of reasons object to having their pictures taken. It is therefore necessary to include the intention to photograph element in the explanations that accompany the informed consent release. Although taking pictures of people in public spaces without their permission used to be a staple of unobtrusive research, such activity now occupies something of a gray ethical area. It is unlikely that any researcher would take pictures in a nominally public space where private activities are going on (e.g., a public lavatory); but we simply cannot assume that we know

what people will and will not consider private, so that even at the risk of being more obtrusive than originally planned, it is ethically advisable to get permission first.

The ethical ramifications of the need to protect human subjects in the case of studies involving photography (still or video) have been explored by Clark and Werner (1997) and Werner and Clark (1998). Identities can be readily disguised when the research is rendered primarily in the form of narrative, but photography makes it very easy to identify participants. Techniques used to disguise people's images can perhaps protect their anonymity, but can such deliberately distorted images really represent the social scene as it was observed by the researcher?

It is also worth noting that photographs are not merely functional adjuncts to the research process; they can be aesthetically pleasing—works of art, even, if properly executed in ways that notes jotted on a pad probably never are. We will later consider non-verbal ways of representing research data; an artistically mounted photographic display might well be an effective way of conveying the sense of a particular research setting, even if is not as explicit as a supposedly objective written scientific report. (See Mead and Bateson, 1977 for a revealing debate between two pioneers in the field comparing and contrasting the scientific and the aesthetic value of photography in research.) Digital photography has eliminated some of the problems inherent in printing and preserving photos, but it does raise issues of its own regarding indexing and accessing digital files. As with any other kind of field "note," a photo, whether digitized or not, whether artful or simply functional, should be stored in such a way as to assure the confidentiality of its subjects.

Videotape.

Videotape equipment now makes it possible to capture behavior in motion, an important addition to the repertoire of gesture available to the still camera. Videotaping is a way of reliving the field experience so that observations can be repeated at will in order to discern levels of nuance hidden at the outset. Videotape can also be useful as a training tool by capturing novice workers in action so that their procedures can be discussed with their mentors. Videotaping can now be accomplished with relatively simple and inexpensive equipment that is far less obtrusive than first-generation machines. Most people nowadays are as comfortable with being videotaped as their parents were with being the subjects of "snapshots." The same ethical precautions, however, are in effect with videotape as with still photography; we can never merely assume that it is acceptable to tape, but must always get written permission from subjects after carefully explaining the purposes of the

taping and the ways in which the tape may or may not be used in public presentations. Further, storage of videotaped materials must comply with norms for the preservation of the confidentiality of subjects.

Clips from videotapes can be used to illustrate research reports in multi-media formats, although they tend to be more widely used as aids to the memory of researchers. The repeat viewings of the taped observations are thus subject to note taking in other media; the videotape cannot really stand alone as a conveyor of information. The use of film, as distinct from videotape, has a long history in ethnographic research, but documentary films are almost always representational products of a research project rather than aids to the collection of primary field data. See below for a further consideration of the use of film as representation of data.

Computers.

Computers have been used by researchers to "crunch" data and, of course, to write reports for quite a while now. But the ready availability of laptop and notebook-style computers has now brought computer technology directly to the field site. Many researchers now use them in preference to the trusty old pads and pens when taking notes. Laptops certainly have the advantage of allowing researchers to type their notes directly, without going through the intermediate step of having to decipher written scrawl. But if hiding behind a pad creates barriers to optimal social interaction, how much more off-putting might be a researcher parked behind a keyboard? It is true that in most settings nowadays people are used to seeing laptops; they do not necessarily make researchers more conspicuous than they might otherwise be. But researchers must always be alert to the possibility that their technology is creating distance between them and the people they are observing, particularly in settings in which they are playing a fairly active membership role. In any case, as with any sort of technology, it is important to go into the field fully prepared: Is the equipment in proper order? Do I know how to use it properly? Do I have all the necessary peripherals and back-ups? When considering software, flexibility and user-friendliness should be the main criteria. Before choosing software, researchers should determine whether it is actually designed to perform the task at hand; if not, it is necessary to find out whether it can be adapted to that task or if an alternative must be identified. Researchers should ascertain whether software comes with a readable manual, has on-screen help, and/or has a tech support phone line.

Weitzman and Miles (1995, p. 5) summarize the main tasks associated with fieldwork that might be facilitated by the **use of computers**, including: making notes in the field; writing up or transcribing field notes; editing, correcting, extending, or revising field notes; coding (attaching keywords or tags to segments of text to permit later retrieval); storage (keeping text in organized databases); search and retrieval (locating relevant segments of texts and making them available for inspection); data "linking" (connecting relevant data segments to one another, forming categories, clusters, or networks of information); memoing (writing reflective commentaries on some aspect of the data as a basis for deeper understanding); content analysis (counting frequencies, sequence, or locations of words or phrases); data display (placing selected or reduced data in a condensed organized format, such as a matrix); conclusion-drawing and verification; theory-building; graphic mapping (creating diagrams that depict findings and/or theories); and preparing interim and final reports.

For Discussion

1. Comment on the ways you think the procedures discussed in this chapter can and cannot address the issues of validity and reliability that concern practitioners of observation-based research. Share your insights with an appropriate peer group.

Chapter Five

The Ethics of Naturalistic Observation

The Ethics of Naturalistic Observation

Observation-based social research by definition brings researchers into proximity with the people they are studying. The relationship between researchers and their study populations may be quite intimate, depending on the degree to which one of the more active membership roles is sought out; but even in unobtrusive or non-reactive observational research, the possibility exists that the process of observation may somehow affect the lives of the members of the study group. In our survey of types of observational research, we have seen how opportunities to do harm—even inadvertently—can arise during the process of social research. We must ensure that we understand, and abide by relevant standards for the ethical conduct of research.

Types of Ethical Standards

The field of research ethics is a complex one, as we must be aware that our behavior as researchers is judged against at least three distinct standards. First, we must recognize our own personal values, which may derive from our religious traditions, consensus among our peer groups, family traditions, or our reflections on issues of concern. Second, we may have reference to codes of ethics promulgated by professional societies. For example, the American Anthropological Association (AAA) stipulates (and explains in great detail) that the primary responsibility of researchers is to the *people with whom they work and whose lives and cultures they study*. The AAA certainly recognizes the responsibilities of researchers to scholarship and the scientific community, as well as to the general public, but it gives priority to the relationships that develop between researchers and their study populations. Third, there are official, published standards mandated by the government and operative in universities and other research institutions that accept federal funding. Since the 1960s, the federal government has required such institutions to have in place institutional review boards (IRB's) to monitor the degree to which researchers comply with the accepted canons of **informed consent**. Moreover, principal investigators on IRB-reviewed projects must take annual continuing education courses on evolving federal ethical standards.

Informed Consent and the Protection of Human Subjects

The government first became concerned with the protection of study populations (which are usually referred to in the federal regulatory language guiding IRB's as "human subjects of research") in the wake of several research projects whose intrusive procedures led to the injury or even death of participants. The government response was to make sure that participation in research was a choice that was under the control of potential subjects. In order to make a valid choice, people needed to be informed—in clear, jargon-free language—before the project began about what would be involved and what the aims of the project would be. It is true that the harmful and intrusive research that caught the government's attention was mostly biomedical in nature; the potential of such research to do physical or psychological injury seemed clear. But what of social research? The sad fact is that whenever we insert ourselves into a study community, we have the capacity to disrupt the lives of its members; we can inadvertently cause emotional distress by highlighting sensitive issues or we can change the dynamic of relationships within the community in ways the people might not like.

Confidentiality

Even if subjects understand the study and approve of its goals, they may be leery about what happens to personal, privileged information once researchers go back to their offices to write their papers. The federal guidelines also mandate the use of precautions to safeguard privacy and to maintain the confidentiality of research records. Since we cannot assume that we know which matters people in the study population will consider private, it is necessary to confer with them so that we can spell out appropriate measures to keep information from being shared with anyone not approved by the community. It must be kept in mind, however, that researchers do not share the privilege customarily enjoyed by clergy, physicians, or lawyers; that is, they do not have an automatic privilege of confidentiality. That being the case, our records cannot readily withstand a court subpoena. Like journalists protecting their sources, we can refuse to comply with such a court order; but we pay the consequences if we do so. So part of our confidentiality agreement with subjects must be the disclaimer that while we will do everything in our power to respect and preserve their privacy, there are circumstances under which records might have to be surrendered. Under the principle of informed consent, however, it is up to the potential "human subject" to decide whether or not such limited protection is good enough.

Virtual Ethics

In a later section we will discuss the application of the traditional techniques of naturalistic observation to the brave new world of on-line or virtual reality. A comprehensive ethic of research in virtual communities has not yet been articulated, although the issues have been summarized in a very thorough fashion by Buchanan (2004). At this point it is fair to say that the basic principles of informed consent and the maintenance of confidentiality remain the researcher's overriding concerns, although the technical problems of adhering to such principles when one is not in face-to-face contact with the people one is studying can be quite challenging.

The Review Process

Most social researchers agree that the protections embedded in the current federal standards have indeed made research a more ethical practice. Many, however, are uncomfortable with the assumption that their brand of inquiry is on par with truly intrusive biomedical research. Even the continuing education courses on ethics (which can be taken on-line) offered on a national basis and accepted by all IRB's are all drawn from the area of health services research, rather than social research per se. In partial agreement with that position, the government now allows social researchers to request either an expedited review (or, in cases of research that can be shown beyond a doubt to be "non-reactive," a complete exemption from review) *unless* their human subjects are members of designated **vulnerable populations**, including children, people with disabilities (especially those who are mentally challenged), people in prison, and the elderly. Such people may be impeded in their ability to understand the nature of research, or they may believe that their officially subordinated position does not allow them to make a free choice. Researchers studying such vulnerable populations must therefore take extra precautions to assure informed consent and the protection of confidentiality.

Most IRB's err on the side of caution; even proposals that seem to be exempt (e.g., studies relying on material that has previously been videotaped and is already in a public archive) must still be filed for review. In general, IRB's have become increasingly skeptical about granting exemptions to "non-reactive" research in general. After all, the basic premise of unobtrusive inquiry in which researchers take on the complete observer role as described earlier is that the "human subjects" are *not* informed that research is taking place. Since the possibility exists that harm could befall them anyway, and since they have not been given a chance to give informed consent, this style of research strikes some reviewers as unethical on its face—one reason, perhaps, why it is somewhat out of favor with contemporary social researchers.

Perhaps the most difficult ethical challenge for qualitative researchers in general, and those using observational techniques in particular, is the apparent discontinuity between what IRB's seem to expect and what this brand of research is prepared to deliver. IRB's, reflecting their genesis in the world of biomedical research, are familiar with experimental designs in which variables are carefully controlled and research instruments (interview schedules, observation guides) are prepared in advance, and can be reviewed for potential ethical problems before the research gets underway. However, qualitative field research often develops in unexpected ways; it is not always possible (and is probably not even desirable) for such researchers to enter the field with preplanned instruments and a fully developed checklist of things to do. Their proposals are therefore sometimes rejected by IRB's who find too many ambiguities and openings for unfortunate accidents in them. Some qualitative researchers have responded by rethinking their projects so that they are more nearly "scientific" in their approach. Others have tried to reform the review system itself so that IRB's can appreciate the special circumstances of fieldwork. At my university, for example, there are now two IRB's, one for biomedical research and one for social and behavioral research. This structure has not, however, completely solved the problem as the social and behavioral panel is dominated by psychologists. This alignment is not altogether

unreasonable as the psychology department is by far the biggest in the College of Arts and Sciences at my university. But most psychological research is still conceived in terms of scientific/experimental designs, and its practitioners are not necessarily less baffled than scholars from the natural and physical sciences when it comes to a proposal for qualitative fieldwork. (See Lincoln, 2005 for an extended treatment of this problem.)

The fact is that professional research ethical standards, like any standards, are written in general terms but are then subject to interpretation. Even supposedly explicit laws are subject to judicial review. Each university or other research institution will interpret ethical guidelines in its own way. Some are very strict, preferring to err on the side of caution; they insist on seeing very detailed plans for what the researcher will be doing in the field and lean toward lengthy, legalistically phrased documents for informed consent. The degree of legalistic language does not, alas, prove effective should a research "subject" feel aggrieved after the fact. In the United States, as my university's legal counsel told me, anybody can sue anybody for anything, whether they have a valid case or not. Moreover, some IRB's are relatively lenient and take the broadest possible interpretation of both informed consent and the protection of confidentiality. For example, photos taken in the field generally require explicit written permission in order to be published or used in any form of public presentation; some IRB's, however, will make exceptions for photos taken in public places, so long as individual identities cannot be discerned.

The problem is compounded when one's research involves not only one's home university but another kind of institution with its own IRB structure. My hospital research, for example, had to be approved by both the university and the hospital review panels. I was a little surprised to find that the university was far more restrictive than the hospital. The latter had no problem with my observing the ER and were content to let the Chief of Emergency Medicine sign a blanket release; the only caution was that I was not to use patients' real names, something I did not need to do anyway since the focus of my observation was the interactions among staff. Although it had not occurred to me to take pictures (I just assumed that doing so would be prohibited and so never built it into my research plan) I later found out that there would have

been no objections, as long as I didn't get in anyone's way and, again, as long as no picture could be used to identify a patient. On the other hand, the university IRB was quite insistent on my getting signed releases from every member of the staff; since for obvious reasons I could not get signed statements from patients being treated in the trauma bays, I was not permitted to be in those areas at all for research purposes, although I could go in when no patients were there so that I could map the room, copy the wall charts, and so forth. I suspect that the hospital's relative leniency might have had something to do with the fact that I was already known to the staff from my prior work in pastoral care; it is likely that someone going to the hospital for the first time with a proposal to observe the ER would have been made to satisfy more stringent requirements.

For all these reasons, it is advisable to check with your own institution's IRB to see what it specifically is looking for; consult also with other members of your department to see what standards they were asked to conform to when they submitted successful IRB applications.

Relational Ethics in Context

Compliance with the federal guidelines and codes of professional ethics certainly takes us a long way toward the goal of conducting ethically sound research. But there are still a few problems that we need to take into account. For example, many social researchers take offense at the very label "human subjects," a term that, at best, has definite clinical/experimental connotations and that, at worst, is insultingly de-personalizing. It also reflects a hierarchical view of the research process, implying as it does that people being studied are passive "subjects" of the active agent—the researcher. People who conduct qualitative fieldwork are now more inclined to refer to the people they study as research "partners." (The term "collaborators" is also found in the current literature, although the unpleasant connotations to that word lead some to avoid it.)

Social researchers in the "natural laboratory" of the field, particularly those who adopt one of the more active membership roles, often find that their research plans develop as they go along. As noted in the earlier discussion of the interactionist perspective, researchers are as much involved in relationships as the people under study. In fact, the process of fieldwork is a kind of dialogue between researchers and the communities they study. Regardless of the technical skills researchers bring to a project, they are almost completely dependent on the cooperation and good will of their community partners in research. The informed consent of the latter must therefore be based on more than a simple understanding of what researchers want to do "to" them; they must also understand that they have a say in determining how the research will be conducted, and what will become of the results in the end.

The salient question for ethical social researchers is how to balance the intense interactions that may be part of the research plan with the need to maintain some degree of scholarly objectivity so that the results of the research will be taken seriously. (This question may not be applicable to those who adopt an autobiographical position with regard to their study topic.) The answer is probably context and situation-dependent, rather than one that has a simple, universal answer.

For example, when I was conducting my research in Trinidad, I boarded in the home of a local family; they ultimately came to treat me as part of the family, and I was accepted as such by other members of the community. My entrée into the homes and workplaces of others was facilitated by the fact that I had been accepted by a family widely respected in the Indian community. But of course I was *not* a family member, an Indian, or even a Trinidadian. I was clearly an outsider—certainly a sympathetic outsider who had assumed an active membership role, but it was always important for people to remember that I was there primarily to "write a book" (which is how they understood my scholarly purposes), which made it easier for me to insist on maintaining some distance in certain social situations—something that would have been offensive had I been taken as a total insider.

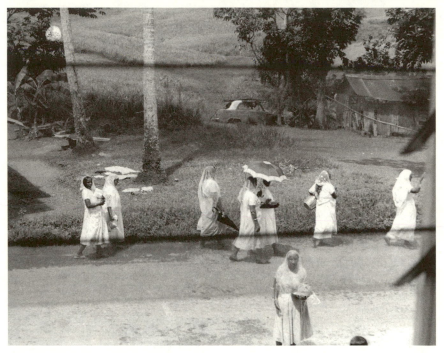

Figure 9: Women on a Village Lane

Describe this scene in as much detail as you can: What do you see? What can you say about the people? About the setting? What do you think is going on? What questions would you like to ask?

I was no less an outsider to the community of adults with mental retardation, but compared with the people in Trinidad, the men in that community were less functionally able to separate my role as their friend from my capacity as someone studying their lives. I could not maintain the same degree of distance that was possible in Trinidad. My writings on the deinstitutionalization research therefore have a far more personal, autobiographical tone than do my other works. These considerations make it more, rather than less, imperative that social researchers pay heed to the nuances of relationships that go beyond the ones formally determined by the official standards of informed consent and the protection of "human subjects." (See Elliott and Stern, 1997; Fluehr-Lobban, 2003; Lipson, 1994; Punch, 1986 for more detailed discussions of the ethics of research.)

For Discussion

1. Return to the proposal for research that you developed in the first section. Discuss the ways in which you would assure compliance with both federally mandated informed consent and protection of human subjects standards and codes of professional conduct relevant to your particular discipline. Also discuss what potential issues of a relational/interaction nature might arise in the course of your research and the ways you propose to deal with them. Present your reflections to an appropriate group of peers, and discuss the similarities and differences in your various approaches.

2. Return to the study you read earlier. What ethical issues emerge from this research? If the author has not explicitly addressed them, what do you imagine they may have been? If you were in the position of the author, what steps would you take to address those issues? Present your reflections to an appropriate group of peers, and discuss the similarities & differences in your various approaches.

Chapter Six

Current Issues in Naturalistic Observation

Current Issues in Naturalistic Observation

Having discussed the basic principles of observation-based field research, we turn our attention to some issues raised earlier that remain sources of debate among practitioners which seem to call for further discussion.

Virtual Observations: Where Is the Field?

People in many parts of the world are spending increasing amounts of time on-line forming **virtual communities**—groups defined by the use of computerized media for communication, rather than by geographic proximity or long-established ties of cultural heritage. While some such communities have been around for a while, many of them are ephemeral in nature, coming into and out of existence as participants' interests and levels of commitment change. Is it possible to translate the techniques of ethnographic observation to the study of virtual communities?

The on-line world as a resource for research.

One observational technique that is very much enhanced on-line is research through **archived materials**. Our ability to use such materials has clearly been improved by methods of digital storage and retrieval, and one has access to vast amounts of stored information available at a keystroke. There will still be interesting and important materials secreted in dusty basements that never get digitized and put on-line, but the internet is clearly a great boon to the researcher needing to delve into both primary and secondary sources on a wide variety of topics.

The on-line world as a study community.

By the same token, one can observe the goings-on in an internet chat room in a way analogous to observations in any other field setting; the chat room is, after all, a natural setting for interaction. It is also, in most cases, a public space, although some virtual communities operate on the basis of formal membership and do not permit casual observers to drop in of their own

accord. It is possible to be unobtrusive while conducting observations in this form of public space, and research based on a content analysis of a public website need not pose any ethical problems. In general, however, the same ethical standards should apply in virtual communities as well as in "real" ones. That is, unobtrusive observations should be carried out only when there is no possibility of anyone being hurt through revelation of identity. Observation based on a more active membership role, by extension, requires researchers to announce their presence, explain their intentions, and in all other respects fulfill the expectations for informed consent. In the interest of preserving confidentiality, researchers should not use real names, e-mail addresses, or any other identifying markers should they publish the results of their research, without explicit permission. Some on-line researchers have adopted the practice of sharing drafts of research reports for comment by members of the virtual community, thereby accomplishing the larger ethical goal of turning "subjects" into empowered "collaborators" in the research process.

Naturalistic observation in the real and virtual worlds.

It is necessary to approach such virtual ethnography with a degree of caution. For one thing, electronic communication is based almost entirely on words or deliberately chosen images. The fieldworker who is used to perceiving behavior through the nuances of gesture, facial expression, tone of voice, and so forth, is at a great disadvantage when working on-line. For that same reason, it is very easy for people communicating on-line to disguise their identities; indeed, sometimes their main purpose in participating in a virtual community is to assume a whole new (and wholly fictitious) identity. Studying the masks people use in social interactions is a time-honored theme of social research, particularly in those aspects influenced by symbolic interactionist theory. But such research has always been predicated on the ability of researchers to use their own observational skills to compare and contrast the use of such facades. When working on-line, it becomes much more difficult to sort out the masks from the reality. (See Hakken, 2003; Markham, 2005; and Miller and Slater, 2000, for more complete discussions of the ethical and methodological challenges of doing ethnographic research on-line.)

Even leaving aside the complications involved in the addition of virtual communities to the roster of settings in which observational research can be conducted, we are left with some interesting questions about what we mean by doing "field" work in the modern world. Ethnographic researchers are beginning to question whether our traditional understanding of our "natural laboratory" holds up under current circumstances.

Just as it was once assumed that we observed and described an objectively real set of details that had an enduring existence whether or not we studied them, field researchers typically believed that the field was simply any "place" (defined geographically or in terms of common interests, as the case might be) where ethnographers carried out observational research and other data collection techniques. Like the behaviors we were supposed to observe, the field itself was a reality that existed apart from the research act. Nowadays, however, our propensity to think of behavior as mediated and interpreted by our presence as observers leads us to think of "the field" as something constructed for the purposes of-and, indeed, in the very act of-conducting research. As Atkinson (1992, p. 9) notes, the field is not a pre-existing phenomenon that we "discover" in order to study it; rather, it is produced in the course of the social transactions in which the researcher participates.

A field "site" is not bounded in a fixed and specific way; rather, it is defined as "the outcome of what the ethnographer may encompass in his or her gaze; what he or she may negotiate with hosts and informants; and what the ethnographer omits and overlooks as much as what the ethnographer *writes*" (Atkinson, 1992, p. 9). In some cases, researchers may even be said to *create* a community by virtue of choosing to study certain people and implying that the links they perceive among the elements of the communities they study are treated as if they were objectively real, rather than the products of abstract analysis. The creation of the field has historically involved both "displacement" (which typically meant leaving "home" to study some place that could be defined as different from home, even if it only meant crossing to the other side of town) and the application of "focused, disciplined attention" by means of learning the local language, engaging in systematic observation, and attending to the meanings involved in behaviors (Clifford, 1997, p. 186). These processes have resulted in the exaggeration of differences between "us" and "others," and has fostered the (misleading) idea that what we observe when we get "there" is

somehow a set of "natural" acts that would have gone on even without our presence. According to Gupta and Ferguson (1997, p. 37) fieldwork is more properly thought of as "a self-conscious shifting of social and geographic location," or perhaps "a form of motivated and stylized dislocation" that serves to enhance researchers' sensitivity to other ways of life.

The traditional notions of "the field" as a geographic place derive from the classic cultural and social anthropologists (both American and British) of the early twentieth century. But as powerful and seductive as this image has always been, there have always been dissenters. For example, in the ethnomethodological tradition, the "field" is defined as "wherever reality-constituting interaction takes place" (Gubrium and Holstein, 1997, p. 52). The postmodernist critique, which explicitly disavows the link between "the field" and fixed location, is but the most recent example of questions that have always existed about the reality of the laboratory that we would like to think of as "natural." Malkki (1996, p. 92), for example, discusses "accidental communities of memory," which might include people who have experienced war together, survivors of some sort of disaster, people who suffer from a common illness, or people who participated in a community project. In all of these cases, it is the communities that can be considered "accidental," not the experiences themselves.

Observer Bias

Qualitative researchers in general, and those who use observational techniques in particular, have long been vulnerable to charges that their findings are **biased** because of the subjectivity that is an inevitable part of this style of inquiry. This problem was taken quite seriously in the days when it was assumed uncritically that social research had to conform to the standards of objectivity and value-neutrality that characterize the natural and physical sciences. Observational researchers therefore insisted that they could mitigate bias by making sure that they were introduced to the community by widely trusted and respected gatekeepers. This was intended to lead to a situation in which the presence of the researchers was not a matter of concern; people would go about their business as if the stranger in their midst were just an

ordinary part of the scenery. Moreover, they pointed out that they used triangulation to make sure that they were not simply getting the results they started out looking for; using multiple sources for data collection meant that any bias that might have crept into one kind of research encounter would be compensated for by the application of other ways of approaching the data.

If these arguments seem a little hollow, it is probably because they really are not very convincing. For one thing, as we have already seen, gatekeepers— even ones with impeccable reputations in their communities—are not, and cannot be, completely disinterested bystanders. Their agendas (whatever they may be, and even if they are ones endorsed by the majority of the community) inevitably are attached to the researchers they sponsor. Moreover, unless researchers have adopted the complete-observer role (and, for reasons discussed earlier, they are increasingly unlikely to have done so) their presence cannot go unnoticed. They are interacting with people and are, to one degree or another, likely to be participating members of the community they are studying. The presumed objective neutrality of the experimenter behind one-way glass in a controlled laboratory setting simply cannot be duplicated by any researcher in the field where being inconspicuous enough so as not to influence the people one is encountering is usually not a strategy for doing effective fieldwork. In addition, the use of triangulation might well mean that researchers have taken the trouble to amass a convincing body of evidence in support of their findings, but in and of itself it is no guarantee that all the methods employed were not equally structured in such a way as to guarantee certain desired outcomes.

Presence and action as biasing factors.

When carrying out fieldwork in living communities (as distinct from conducting experiments in the laboratory setting), researchers have always had to factor in the possibility that even if their own methods were pure, their very presence could be a biasing factor: people were reacting to them in ways that took them beyond what they would normally do in the absence of the observer. In addition to this relatively benign distortion, there exists the very real possibility that some members of the study community deliberately deceive researchers, either because they want to make themselves look good (or make their rivals look bad), because they misunderstand the nature and

purposes of research, or simply out of malice or the desire to have a joke at the expense of the nave outsider. It is next to impossible to weed out all these possible distortions and deceptions in the futile hope of stripping the setting back to its "natural" purity. In fact, if one is aware that one is not being dealt with "honestly," then it is possible to make the deception itself the subject of investigation. When people deceive, either deliberately or unintentionally, they are still telling a story—one that is full of cultural meaning. Even if the manifest content of what they do or say is somehow falsified, there is still truth in the way they go about communicating with the deceived researcher and hence establishing a relationship in terms that make sense in their own social world. Indeed, in both my monastery and deinstitutionalization studies, I made extensive use of the way in which my informants chose to misrepresent themselves to me as clues to the ways in which relationships were initiated and sustained in those communities.

Is social research ever value-free?

It may be pertinent to point out that the experimental setting is one in which researchers explicitly control the variables; can we be absolutely certain that they are not also sometimes guilty of **stacking the deck** so as to come up with the results they had projected? This is not the place to consider such issues with regard to quantitative research, but it does put the supposed problem of observer bias in a more inclusive context. Indeed, nearly five decades ago prominent social scientists were questioning the assertion that *any* social research was, could be, or even should be value-free (Gouldner, 1962). In our own time, various schools of social theory as noted earlier have openly embraced subjectivity, tossing aside the cult of objectivity as an artifact of a scientific model that, vital as it is in the study of the physical universe, is simply inappropriate to the study of human social behavior. It is now less common than it once was to hear social researchers claim to be striving for "value-free" or "value-neutral" research. It is now clearly recognized that values define and shape all forms of research. "Observation," say Schensul, Schensul, and LeCompte (1999, p. 95), "is always filtered through the researcher's interpretive frames." Even if a formal research hypothesis derives from a body of abstract theory, it is the researcher's choice to find one school of theory more compelling than another. That choice may be guided by objective, scientific criteria, but the researcher is still taking a value-laden

stance, proposing in effect that one set of ideas is better than another. When dealing with social research based on questions or propositions derived from an interest in current events and conducted with intent to influence public policy or the delivery of social services, then the research is by definition value-explicit. Again, the selection of a social issue, the choice of an explanatory model, and the advocacy of certain recommendations may all be guided by principles that are themselves defined objectively—but the element of choice is still there. If the world were full of self-evident truths, there would be no need for research at all; that the world is full of ambiguity means that our decisions about what is important enough to study and how best to understand and make real-world decisions about those issues reflect subjective judgment. Lumping all such necessary subjective judgments into a category negatively described with the title "bias" does not serve the best interests of the research community.

Subjective judgment.

It goes without saying that there are some unethical researchers whose research really *is* biased for all the wrong reasons. But our concern here is with the kinds of subjectivity that are part of research undertaken using sound data collection techniques and that is in conformity with current ethical standards. In that context, we are learning how to be more consciously aware of the **sources of our subjective judgment**—not to eliminate them entirely, but to use them so that they enhance rather than obscure the research endeavor.

Ethnocentrism.

Ethnocentrism is the tendency to think that one's own way of doing and thinking about things is inherently the best, most logical, and most advanced. Anthropologists, particularly those of the Boasian school of American historical particularism as discussed earlier, were in the forefront of the move to rid social science of its ethnocentric biases in favor of a culturally relativistic approach to the comparative study of human social behavior. Versions of that relativistic stance are now commonly accepted throughout the social sciences. After all, there does not seem to be much point in studying a community that you are convinced is somehow inferior to your own; one has already reached a conclusion and so the only thing to be done is to collect information designed to support that conclusion. Doing so would be an act of pure research bias.

But what corrective is really applied by the adoption of a relativistic stance? For one thing, it is important to keep in mind that cultural relativism is not the same as moral relativism; a researcher who comes across things like domestic violence, exploitation of children, substance abuse, unequal treatment before the law of women and minorities, and so forth, is certainly not obliged to endorse such practices. Just because such things happen in the world does not mean that they all have an equivalent moral value. But our first job as researchers is to find out how such things play out in their social contexts: What is really going on, and why do people behave in this way? To say that we must understand such practices in their proper **cultural and social context** (the essential meaning of cultural relativism) is not to say that we agree that these things are all okay. ("The Yanomamo beat their wives—why shouldn't we?") In fact, any social researcher with any sort of applied agenda is tacitly admitting that some things are wrong and need to be changed. But it is only possible to reach a reasonable decision about what to do by first understanding what is going on in context, and this we can only do by setting aside our ethnocentric preconceptions of proper social behavior.

We may well agree that female circumcision, for example, is wrong for all sorts of reasons that involve moral, legal, and public health concerns; but we will get nowhere by simply preaching against it unless we understand how and why the practice has survived for centuries in certain cultures. Our distaste for the practice may lead us to label it "genital mutilation" and make us want to "do something" about it; but if we act solely on that distaste, without due appreciation for the historical factors that gave rise to the practice and to the sociocultural factors that support and sustain it, we are unlikely to make much of an impact. (See Gruenbaum, 2001 for a review of the female circumcision controversy and its relationship to the principle of cultural relativism in social research.) Social researchers may sometimes adopt the causes espoused by social reformers or even missionaries, but it is our cultural relativism that enables us to bring more than moral fervor to the table. Research on a topic like female circumcision could hardly be "value free." But embracing a value-explicit position and eschewing "neutrality" is not the same thing as surrendering at least some aspects of scientific objectivity.

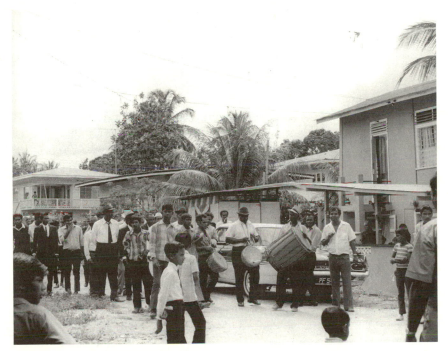

Figure 10: A Wedding Scene

What does this photo suggest about the nature of Hindu weddings in Trinidad? Describe the scene in as much detail as you can. What can you say about the participants and their relationship to one another? What can you observe about the setting in which they are interacting?

The real problem for us as researchers is that ethnocentrism is not such an easy thing to put on a back burner. It is a very natural—and, in some contexts, a quite admirable—human quality. It seems clear that most humans naturally gravitate toward those who seem most like themselves. They tend to form enduring social groups with others who look and act and think more or less like they do. Even in the virtual communities of cyberspace where it is impossible to judge people on their physical characteristics, membership is still essentially a matter of affinity—people continue to participate to the extent that they feel supported in their interest in a certain movie or game or other activity. That feeling of comfort with "one's own kind" is, in and of itself, a benign aspect of "human nature," and to the extent that it contributes to the stability and cohesion of social groups, it may be said to have a positive effect. Trouble enters the picture when this benign preference for the comfort of communities of likeness turns into a distrust of, a disdain or disregard for, or

even a malignant hatred of people who look and act and think differently. This form of ethnocentrism is disruptive of the social order in general, and it is destructive of the research endeavor in particular.

Situatedness and social research.

An important element in the postmodernist challenge to the scientism of traditional social research has been its insistence that we are all prisoners of our own "situations," which include most prominently our race, social class, and gender, as well as our sexual orientation, age category, and degree of disability (Haraway, 1998). In effect, we project onto the world we study the preconceptions emanating from our own particular situations; the postmodernists claim that much of what we have come to think of as objective history or sociology or psychology is really a reflection of the point of view of an elite segment of the population, namely affluent white males. The overall project of postmodernism is to unpack our received assumptions about the world, to relieve them of the encumbrances of that traditional affluent white male situation, and to open up the discourse to alternative, heretofore marginalized voices. In effect, the postmodernist critique involves not so much a call to set aside the factors of our respective situations that may predispose us to think ethnocentrically as it is a reminder that we must be conscious of those factors and so be less arrogant in claiming universal truth-value to observations and conclusions that are, in fact, radically "situated." Whether or not one buys into the postmodernist program in its entirety, it is difficult to escape the conclusion that the genie is out of the bottle, never to be put back in its entirety. We are now conscious of the predispositions we carry with us into our own research and are much more likely to pay attention to the possibility of such predispositions in the work of others.

It is sometimes assumed that photography is a way of minimizing the bias inherent in ethnographic fieldwork because, after all, "pictures don't lie." But pictures do not take themselves; someone has to choose what to shoot, how and when to shoot it, how to edit it, how to use it in some sort of representational product. "The camera," as Lincoln and Denzin (2003, p. 240) note, "is an ideological tool. It represents reality in a particular way, including a way that hides the observer's presence." So photography, an important aid to observational fieldwork, is not immune to the questions about ethnocentrism, situatedness, and value-explicitness that surround observational research in general.

One result of this shift in perspective has been a recognition that the world does indeed speak to us in many voices; truth, it may be said, is **multivocalic**. We cannot realistically strive to achieve a universally accepted, objective, value-neutral "truth"; rather, we should strive to blend our voices, in full recognition of the situations from whence they emanate, in order to establish a kind of mosaic view that approaches—although never quite achieves— absolute "truth."

Situational Attributes: Further Considerations

The preceding section highlighted a shift among social researchers toward a heightened consciousness of the situational factors that are important determinants of their research. Two of those attributes, **race/ethnicity** and **gender**, have been studied in some detail by researchers trying to enhance their understanding of their own processes.

Race and ethnicity.

In common parlance, "ethnicity" is generally taken to mean a social category based on shared culture, while race is a social category rooted in biological characteristics. It is now generally accepted in the scientific community that race really has no standing as a biological or genetic category; explicating the reasons behind this conclusion are far beyond the scope of this book, but they are carefully summarized with a minimum of scientific jargon by Diamond (2003). Nevertheless, race persists as a social status—in many ways, the pre-eminent one in the United States. Even though the factors we commonly use to define racial identity (e.g., skin color, shape of nose, texture of hair) are virtually useless as biogenetic demarcations of group identity, they have been used most effectively throughout history as excuses to treat certain people differentially. When groups are identified as "different" and are treated unequally, it is only to be expected that they will develop a sense of themselves as a people set apart; they will have a strong sense of collective identity, particularly if they see themselves as having been the victims of persecution and oppression, and that sense is so powerful that it might as well be the result of biology.

In terms of observational research, the *perceived* ethnic or racial category to which a researcher belongs is often of major importance when it comes to site selection, gaining entrée, establishing rapport, and carrying out a project. To be sure, there are cases where there may be little or no effect. In studying the monastery, for example, the fact that I am of Italian ethnic heritage hardly mattered, since some of the monks were also Italian, while others came from German, Polish, French Canadian, and Mexican backgrounds. For the monks, the fact that I had been raised a Catholic and was familiar with Catholic culture was far more important than my ethnicity in their decision to accept me temporarily into their community. By the same token, in studying a big-city hospital emergency room, which typically features a large and widely diverse staff, neither my race nor my ethnic background has ever come up. My acceptance depends solely on having some professional credibility to be in the ER in the first place. And in studying the Southern Anthropological Society, a group of professionals who wouldn't be caught dead categorizing a fellow researcher on the basis of his race or ethnicity, all that mattered was that I was a certified member of the club.

On the other hand, more typical are those situations in which these matters cannot, and do not go unnoticed. In Trinidad, for example, my Italian ethnicity was irrelevant, but my being perceived as white was crucial. At the time I began my study there, the Indian community was vocally insistent on differentiating itself from the black (locally referred to as "creole") segment of the population. It was very important to the Indians' self-image that they not be confused with the creoles, whose ancestors had been slaves and who had come from Africa, a place lacking in ancient civilization (or so they thought). The outside observer might point out that the indenture had reduced the Indians to a condition economically and socially indistinguishable from slavery (albeit for a time-limited period), but to the Indians the difference had to be upheld. Moreover, they knew that European scholars had long been fascinated by the glories of Indian philosophy, religion, and art, and so they saw themselves as linked to the colonial master class in a way that most definitely did not encompass the creole descendents of slaves. My decision to study their community was seen as a validation of their self-image, that theirs was a culture worthy of the attention of a white person from North America. (At that point many of them were still sufficiently isolated so that they did not realize that many white North Americans and Europeans had studied the creoles of Trinidad and other parts of the West Indies. Those who knew told

me that such studies were akin to biologists "looking at bugs under a microscope," whereas a study like mine was more a matter of my desire to be uplifted and enlightened by what I learned about their world view.)

Although my complexion might enable me to "pass" as an Indian in a pinch, I soon learned that it for the members of the community it was essential that I not do so. I was more valuable to them as a white person who had *chosen* to live among them for an extended period of time. One of the advantages of traditional anthropological fieldwork is that a researcher is on site for an extended period of time, and I believe that by the end of my first thirteen-month visit I had become a familiar enough presence so that I was accepted (or rejected, as the case might be) just as myself, and not as a representative of the entire white race paying homage to Indian civilization. But for the first two or three months I was unable to shake the feeling that I was being treated as an honored guest rather than a real down-among-the-people participant observer.

Whenever I have conducted fieldwork in the West Indies I have experienced some of what I have heard "people of color" say about being in the minority in North America—that they feel as if they are being constantly stared at. In the context of the West Indies in the late 1960s and early 1970s, however, whatever feelings might have been in play beneath the surface, those stares were expressed through a surface of deference and respect. I was often addressed (sometimes with evident irony, but usually not) as "Captain," an old plantation term for the white field boss. I suppose it is better to be treated with respect (even if grudgingly offered) than with hostility, but being the object of deference is almost as damaging to good fieldwork as being scorned, since it means that honest human relationships are foreclosed. I had to work very hard, once I belatedly caught on to the problem, to make sure that I was treated as an individual and not as a representative of a perceived racial category.

Insider research.

If perceived racial/ethnic difference can be a hindrance to fieldwork, perceived insider status is no guarantee of success. To be sure, there are advocates of "insider research" conducted by scholars who share the race and/or ethnicity of the community under study. (See, e.g., Zavella, 1996). But others are more skeptical (e.g., Zinn, 1979), fearing that calls for group "loyalty" could undermine the cause of objective research. It is one thing to consciously choose to be an advocate for one's ethnic community; it is another

to be assumed to want to—or to have to—play that role by other members of the racial/ethnic community who would see it as a betrayal to do otherwise. Moreover, even researchers who share an identity with the community under study are still separated from them by the very fact that they are there temporarily and for the very specific purpose of conducting research. They are rarely in a position to become "full participants" of the community to the extent that people might like or expect them to be, at least for the duration of the research project.

For field researchers, there are always two crosscutting factors at work: race/ethnicity as they choose to identify themselves, and race/ethnicity as a category attributed to them through the perceptions of others. Negotiating these boundaries in an area as historically fraught with conflict and tension as race relations is a tricky matter even in everyday life—although presumably in everyday life we can choose to absent ourselves from situations in which these issues might come to the fore. But if we choose to insert ourselves into research sites whose members will not let us set those issues aside, then we have to learn to be creative in incorporating those tensions into the conduct of research. For example, Duneier (1994), a white researcher, conducted a field study centered around the activities of an African American street person named Hasan. Over the years, the two developed a good working relationship; Hasan even co-taught a course with Duneier and contributed an appendix to his book. Duneier says that he never tried to undo the perception that he was an "outsider" (perhaps by self-consciously adopting the language, clothing styles, and body language of an urban African American); rather, he used his outsider status to identify by contrast various features of the world of the street that was his research site. He saw himself as a kind of one-man control group; he compared the way he was treated in particular situations to the way other kinds of people were treated on the street. As Liebow (1967, p. 251) noted with regard to his own study of black street-corner society, "...the wall between us remained, or better, the chain-link fence.... When two people stand up close to the fence on either side, without touching it, they can look through the interstices and forget that they are looking through a fence."

Gender.

Just as many people consider race to be a biological category, so do many think of gender as a genetically determined attribute. Social scientists are nowadays inclined to make a nuanced distinction between sex, the physical expression of genetically inherited characteristics- particularly those related to

the biological function of reproduction -and gender, the set of behaviors and other learned characteristics that are considered to be culturally appropriate manifestations of sex. Sexuality, or sexual orientation, is the set of choices that people make about how to use their biological attributes; it is largely independent of both sex and gender. The precise relationship between genetics and socialization in this area is very complex and is by no means a settled matter; however, the current consensus is that what we consider to be appropriate behavior for a man or for a woman has little to do with underlying biology and a great deal to do with social and cultural expectations. (See Kottak and Kozaitis, 2003, pp. 142-159 for a useful summary of these issues.)

Our own culture leads us to think that because there are two biological sexes, then there must be two, and only two dichotomously defined genders, male and female. And we have very definite, albeit stereotyped views as to what constitutes proper male and female behavior and the roles they may play in society at large; at least until very recently, the assumption was that doctors were men and nurses were women because men were naturally authoritative and good at mastering complex scientific skills while women were naturally nurturing and caring. But just as race is not a matter of absolute "black" and "white" categories, but rather is a continuum of shades, so gender is best thought of as being expressed in a wide range of possible behaviors. By the same token, society at large tends to resist these insights gained through social science and continues to assign people to supposedly mutually exclusive gender categories (and gets upset when people do not conform) just as they continue to attribute racial categories even in an increasingly pluralistic world. For researchers, this tension echoes that involved in race/ethnicity; the gender we are *perceived* to belong to must be negotiated against the specific behaviors and roles we adopt for ourselves. And we must keep in mind the possibility that behaviors and roles that are considered perfectly within the "normal" range (whatever that means) in our own culture might be considered suspiciously inappropriate elsewhere. For example, despite our culture's rigidity about some aspects of male and female domestic roles, it has always been acceptable for men to cook—the profession of chef being an honorable one, particularly in certain ethnic groups. In my own case, I like to cook and at least a few of the people I have cooked for have lived to tell the tale. But among the Indians of Trinidad thirty years ago, the very idea of a man cooking dinner was bizarre in the extreme. The lady in whose house I boarded was shocked but amused when we watched a TV cooking show and I said I would be happy to cook dinner for the family some time before I left. She took me up on my offer, and seemingly half the village gathered outside her kitchen window to

watch this remarkable exhibition. I am sure I did not inspire the village's men to make a mad rush to take up their wives' pots and pans, and I suspect that they chalked up my proclivities to some sort of unfathomable North American affectation. But even at that early stage of my career I knew better than to push the envelope with some sort of misguided "natural experiment," perhaps wearing jewelry and a sari while I cooked just to gauge the reaction.

Our culture has historically been dominated by the male perspective and so whenever social scientists endeavored to study other people in other societies with different cultures, they automatically assumed that the male view would be the only one worth recording. Although a few pioneering women social scientists such as Margaret Mead made a point of incorporating observations of female activities into their studies of other cultures, the perspectives of half of humanity were conspicuously absent until the advent of a formal feminist ideology that came into academic prominence in the 1970s. A good deal of the first generation of feminist social science was dedicated to the recovery of "women's roles" in the larger picture of society and culture. More recently, feminist scholarship has turned to a consideration of gender in more general terms: how is it defined in a particular community? what effect does it have on relations among the people? how does it shape access to power and other resources? (See Warren, 2001 for a review of the evolution of feminist approaches to field research.)

It is probably worth mentioning in this context that Mead's groundbreaking study in Samoa was criticized after her death by Derek Freeman, who complained that Mead had missed the main point of Samoan culture because she did not (or could not) have access to the male chiefs. It is certainly true that Mead focused on the young women and tended to view the entire culture through their experiences. It is also true that Freeman has done some fine fieldwork on the male/chiefly side of things. But it is ironic that Freeman seems to assume that the male view is somehow more real or more salient than the female and that by focusing on the women, Mead was somehow distorting the truth of Samoan culture. Surely the truth of any culture is that men and women somehow forge workable relationships of some sort; good ethnography should somehow endeavor to encompass those mutual relationships. But the preconceptions of our culture, with its well-established gender dichotomy, lead even well trained social scientists to think that the entire world must function in ways that mirror our own standards when it comes to this intensely personal, profoundly contested area of gender. (Freeman makes a number of additional points in his critique of Mead; I have,

however, emphasized the matter of gender difference since it is most pertinent to the issues addressed in this section. See Holmes, 1986 for a reasonably even-handed analysis of the Mead-Freeman controversy.)

There is still a tendency on the part of female fieldworkers to choose to spend the bulk of their time with women and in whatever spheres of activity women are found in various study communities. In many circumstances, this means that they have become students of the domestic arena, particularly with regard to issues surrounding child-rearing, since this is the aspect of social life that so often defines "women's roles." Some women researchers, however, are exploring the worlds of men, deliberately playing on the difference in perspective in the same way that Duneier used racial difference in his study.

An awareness of gender, however, is not restricted to women scholars. Historically, men have not studied women because they did not think women's experiences were worth bothering about; nowadays, they may realize that women's roles are indeed worthy of attention, but they are reluctant to do such research because of perceived taboos against gender interactions. Those taboos are, of course, culturally highly variable. In the early years of my Trinidad study, it was true that I did not have easy access to women of my own age. However, I was semi-formally adopted into the family I was living with, to the extent that the lady of the house took to introducing me to her friends as "just like my own sons." That being the case, I had access to the older women of the village (who, as I found out, really ran the show behind the scenes) in a way that did not threaten anyone's ideas of propriety. But there are certainly some potential field sites that are absolutely dependent on gender perceptions; no woman researcher, no matter how technically expert or personally persuasive, would have been allowed to have been a participant observer in the monastery. By the same token, there is nothing I could have done to have persuaded the powers that be that I would be an appropriate researcher to do a participant observational study of a convent of nuns. Redfern-Vance's (1999) study of military women who were victims of sexual abuse could not have been done with as much success by a male researcher. In mixed-gender communities, some researchers have tried to bridge the gap in gender perception by bringing a spouse or significant other of the other perceived gender into the field, each to interact with people of their own gender. Others object to such a strategy, believing it to reify a gender dichotomy to which they have strong political objections.

As with researchers who are "insiders" because of race/ethnicity, those who are perceived to be part of the group because of their gender are pulled in two directions. On the one hand, they may have a relatively easy time gaining acceptance because they are "just like us." On the other hand, people in the community might expect that they really should behave "just like us" in all respects and so feel some sense of betrayal when researchers put their research agenda ahead of their assumed loyalties to their gender-mates. Just as feminist researchers are sometimes disappointed to find that women in the Third World do not respond to the implicit call of sisterhood (see, e.g., Behar, 1993), so too gay and lesbian researchers have come to learn that "there is no 'universal gay community'" (Lang, 1996, p. 103) so that even when they conduct research among gay people in a setting different from their own, they cannot assume that they will be welcomed uncritically. Lang, who is herself openly gay, conducted research on lesbians but found it unacceptable to begin her observations and her search for informants in bars or other obvious meeting places, since she feared that the other women would assume she was looking for sexual partners. In this case, she decided that identifying herself only as an "ethnographer" would be the best strategy, even though her personal sexual orientation was not at all irrelevant to the theme of the study. Her decision was a strategic one, dictated by her reading of the expectations of the people she proposed to study.

Moreover, race/ethnicity and gender can come into conflict as perceptual categories (Riessman, 1987, p. 179–188). For example, is a white female researcher more or less likely to be able to bond with a study community of African American women as compared with an African American male researcher? In such situations, the social, interactive dynamics that are at play in a particular community must be analyzed before any decisions are made—we cannot assume that all communities are alike just because they share the same demographic attributes. The point is that no one of is just one thing; when asked to define our identities, we rarely, if ever reduce it to a single demographic factor or social category. It is therefore probably unreasonable to assume that we can pick just one thing as the staff on which to hang the flag of our identity while doing fieldwork as members of one sort or another of a study community (Blackwood, 1995, p. 70). We might well have to become "emotionally aware inter-actors engaged with other actors" (Gearing, 1995, p. 211) which means that our identities grow and develop naturally in the course of participating in a study community.

Sexuality and sexual orientation.

The question of gender relations inevitably leads to questions about sexuality. Social researchers certainly include sexual relations among legitimate topics of inquiry, but in the case of researchers who have adopted some sort of membership role in the communities they study, sex is more than simply a matter of objective, clinical interest. An important part of membership-based observational fieldwork is the status of the researcher as a real, identifiable human being who interacts with other human beings. Whether or not we want to think about it, the expression of sex is part of the package. Researchers working on topics that have little to do with sex may be able to avoid the issue; since they are not bringing it up with members of the community, they can expect not to be questioned about it in return. If the research is of a short-term nature, and/or if a researcher is accompanied by a spouse or significant other, questions again may be set aside. But in situations where lone researchers insert themselves as members of a society for a relatively long period of time, questions certainly do arise—not only on the part of curious members of the community, but also in the minds of the researchers themselves. It must be kept in mind that it is certainly valid to choose to be celibate and avoid embarrassing or even dangerous entanglements while in the field. But if such a choice does not fit into a community's expectations about how people behave, it must be carefully explained.

Fieldworkers of all sexual orientations have faced the problem of either becoming sexually involved while in the field (which might compromise objectivity in ways that even a postmodernist might question) or abstaining (which might lead people in the community to wonder about them all the more, making them as people and not their research the objects of attention). This dilemma, once only whispered about in private, has been increasingly brought forward in discussions of fieldwork. Gay and lesbian researchers have perhaps been habituated to concealment, but there is a growing consensus that it is usually better to be forthright; if the proposed research community is uncomfortable with or hostile to homosexuality, it is best to find out right away and make alternative plans.

It is impossible to legislate—let alone enforce—a single standard of appropriate behavior. Researchers' own ethical and moral senses must be their primary guides. Prudence, however, would seem to suggest that whatever researchers choose to do about expressing their sexuality while in the field, they should see to it that their behavior is consonant with the values and norms of the community they are studying, that they do not take advantage of their position (as prestigious and probably relatively wealthy and influential outsiders) to exploit local people, that they do not lead themselves or others into situations that might prove embarrassing or dangerous, and that they do not end up drawing attention to themselves in ways that might disrupt the more or less "normal" course of activities in the "natural laboratory." Looking on the bright side, Altork (1995, p. 132) suggests that "perhaps by acknowledging our own feelings and desires, we might actually look at other people and places more objectively, by being able to ferret out our own biases and distortions as we do our work." (For a variety of analyses of the role of sexuality in fieldwork see Kulick and Willson, 1995; Lewin and Leap, 1996; Whitehead and Conaway, 1986.)

One disturbing, but instructive account of the problems associated with expressing sexuality in the field is that of Moreno (1995), who describes being raped while conducting fieldwork in Ethiopia. She consciously avoided maintaining the "fiction" of a "genderless self" (1995, p. 246), but when a researcher chooses to express her own sexuality, she must always be aware of the degree to which she makes herself the object of attention of others who may see her as a target of sexual advances. Moreno suspects that her attacker was motivated as much by hostility against her status as a "foreign expert" (a category that was being pointedly vilified in the local media at the time) as by sexual desire. Nevertheless, she concludes that "women must always, everywhere, deal with the spectre of sexual violence" (1995, p. 248). It is certainly not inconceivable that sexual violence could be directed against a male researcher, but as a general rule this is a problem of relatively greater concern to women. Moreno points out that it would be a foolish female indeed who stepped into a field setting without having some sense of the sexual mores of the society and who did not plan ahead and take precautions when it came to presenting herself in that setting. It may bear parenthetical notice that "Eva Moreno" is a pseudonym; despite the candor with which she writes about her experience, this scholar is not yet comfortable with full disclosure— a reflection of the sexual mores of our own culture as translated into the field setting.

Description: Thick or Otherwise

As noted earlier, field researchers use naturalistic observation in order to produce descriptions of settings and events and the people who interact within them. Prior to the postmodernist revolution discussed in the previous section, it was generally assumed that ethnographic description involved "stable 'real objects' that can be straightforwardly observed and recorded because they possess inherent meanings" (Emerson, 2001, p. 28). A trained observer was supposed to record and report on these realities in an objective manner. Moreover, since these realities have fixed meanings, two observers of the same phenomenon should come up with the same descriptions; if not, one or the other of them had to be "wrong." By the same token, it was taken for granted that trained observers could, in fact, record every aspect of a setting or event and some of the procedures discussed earlier were explicitly designed to maximize minutely detailed precision. With postmodernist skepticism in mind, these assumptions are no longer automatically accepted. That being the case, what can we now make of the field researcher's basic function of observing and describing?

The current near-consensus among qualitative researchers is that the objective description of the physical surface of behavior, while a good starting point, is insufficient in and of itself. Researchers are now expected to concern themselves with the meanings attached to behavior, meanings that are not necessarily fixed or universally shared within the interacting community. Led by the influential anthropological theorist Clifford Geertz, there are now many social researchers who see their main task as one of "interpretation." Geertz (1973) popularized the philosophical term **thick description** as a way of orienting this interpretive task. Thick description does not mean piling on vivid adjectives. Rather, it refers to a way of depicting a setting or event as seen through the eyes of those participating in it so as to discern the structures of meaning through which people produce, perceive, and interpret their own and others' actions. So while it is still necessary to collect detailed observations, they should in no way be construed as "facts" or "data" that have any reality apart from the meanings the people in the setting affix to them. A fully realized interpretive ethnography, grounded in thick description of settings and events, is the researcher's own imaginative rendering of the meanings that impel the "actors" in the social drama. In Geertz's view, the settings and events that a researcher observes are ephemeral; it is only when they are "inscribed" (reproduced in written or other communicative format) that they achieve some sort of permanent reality. As such, the culture of a community is inseparable from the texts that are produced to represent them. In that sense, the descriptions may seem to be emic but since they must necessarily pass

through the interpretive lens of the researcher in order to become usable "facts," they cannot be said to be directly equivalent to insiders' views. In sum, "descriptions... are not simply *about* some social world but are also *part* of that world" (Emerson, 2001, p. 37).

Membership roles reconsidered.

These considerations have led to a reassessment of the old "membership role" model. An important part of the rationale for assuming a membership role in the study community, as distinct from observing it in some supposedly unobtrusive manner, was that researchers could thereby come to assimilate the "insider's perspective." But a Geertzian emphasis on interpretation would suggest that field researchers and the people they study do not inhabit the same perceptual space; if their worlds came to be completely isomorphic, there would be no need for interpretation in the first place. As Bittner (1973) has pointed out, researchers almost always come into field settings in which they have not grown up. (Even indigenous researchers studying their own communities have probably gone away for training and are thus entering a situation in which they have not been continuously participating.) Researchers' memberships are typically both temporary and voluntary, conditions that separate them from the people they study, no matter how much empathy they have and how assiduously they work to achieve rapport. Doing observational research in the era of interpretivist ethnography means that researchers will need to become even more aware of themselves as actors, since they can no longer assume that they will automatically slip into a fully-blown replica of the mind-set of the people they study.

The Politics of Fieldwork

Having moved away from the notion of fieldwork as a value-neutral endeavor, social researchers have increasingly sought to understand the political nature of their work. Political considerations certainly attach to the controversies surrounding "situations" such as race/ethnicity and gender; in that sense, we all bring politically charged baggage with us into the field. Political matters also very obviously come into play when we choose to offer our research in service to the agenda of groups or agencies; "applied" research of one sort or another has strong roots among ethnographers (Chambers, 2000). We must also be concerned with the way politics may be implicated in the very process of conducting field research.

Although largely unacknowledged by researchers of past generations, fieldwork has always been conducted in a politicized atmosphere, whether it was "exotic" anthropology carried out under the auspices of colonial authorities, or urban sociology that was dependent on the good will of the local powers-that-be. This situation has become more visible—and, in some ways, more readily contested—in the post-colonial world. Researchers who work outside the U.S. must negotiate a complex collection of new national polities rather than a single overarching colonial authority, and must also be sensitive to the concerns of people in the "developing" world about being studied (and hence possibly exploited) by representatives of the affluent, powerful "First World." By the same token, those whose work is in the U.S. now interface with many groups and communities that have become self-aware, even militantly organized to protect their own interests; having the approval of the local political fixer might no longer carry much weight in communities with a heightened sense of their own empowerment. In both cases, communities have come to expect certain things in return for allowing researchers to participate in their activities, and those expectations might well result in a realignment of the intentions the researchers had when they first conceived of the project.

Fieldwork for whom?

Social scientists as a group are well aware of the fact that they have historically favored research among the poor, the powerless, and the marginalized—the "nuts, sluts, and perverts" highlighted in Liazos' (1975) critique of that research. They have done so out of a well intended desire to learn more about such people and hence to contribute to the betterment of their lot. But their interest may also have had something to do with the fact that such people, being powerless, did not have effective means to stop outsiders from coming into their communities for purposes of study. As such, their research could be characterized as having an unpleasant, unhealthy whiff of voyeurism about it.

Perhaps in reaction, there is now relatively more attention being paid to the call to "study up" (Nader, 1969) by focusing research on elites and on the social institutions (e.g., courts, jails, hospitals) that deal most directly with those "disadvantaged" populations. In doing so, however, they have found that the powerful and privileged do not always fancy being studied, which has, at best, a connotation of condescension and, at worst, the threat of being judged or evaluated. These concerns are, of course, exactly the same as the ones that have

troubled "subaltern" populations all along—but elites are in a better position to bar access to their own inner workings. In studying the ER, for example, I have repeatedly been challenged by authority figures who think that despite—or perhaps even because of—my quasi-insider status at the hospital I will turn my observations into a warts-and-all assessment that will ultimately have negative repercussions. In a situation of serious budgetary constraint, with the several departments of the hospital competing for no longer abundantly available funds, their fear is not altogether unreasonable. I have had to work very hard to demonstrate the relevance of a study of the social structure of an ER to larger theoretical interest in the organization and function of the major institutions of society. I have also made it clear that while I will not turn a blind eye toward things within my area of expertise as a social scientist that I think are amiss (i.e., I cannot and will not comment on the quality of medical and other technical procedures, but might have something to say about the potentially negative effects of the rigid occupational caste stratification which often works against the ideal of ER services being a "team effort") neither will I go out of my way to put negative things in the spotlight. I have the impression (and that is all it is) that I have succeeded in convincing most of the people of the integrity of my intentions, but I certainly cannot dismiss the possibility that some people are responding to me out of a desire to put the best possible face on their activities. I certainly trust that while they are in the midst of caring for a trauma patient they are too occupied with the task at hand to worry about what kind of notes I might be filing away, so that they just go about their business in a "natural" manner—the perennial hope of the observational fieldworker.

It is not just elites who are concerned about using research to burnish their reputations. The successors to the last generation of "nuts, sluts, and perverts" who are currently the objects of researchers' attention are now likely to be organized into consciousness-raised groups with an agenda of gaining a more substantial place in the social order. They may welcome studies that demonstrate their plight, but not to the point where they come off looking like the helpless, hopeless dregs of society. They much prefer research that demonstrates the steps they are taking toward empowerment. Researchers may well endorse the goals of either the elite institutions or the disadvantaged groups they supposedly serve, but most would like, if at all possible, to make sure that it is honest research that feeds into those agendas, and not glossed-over accounts that they have been pressured into producing as the price of being allowed to enter the community or the agency in the first place.

When a community is divided.

Many communities, even those that seem to exhibit a fair degree of harmony, are internally divided, sometimes by broad categories such as race/ethnicity or social class, or by more specific local concerns. Sometimes division is intentionally submerged and even vigorously denied unless some unexpected crisis brings it to the fore. The monastery, for example, wanted to project the image of an earthly version of the peaceable heavenly kingdom. But around the time of my study, one of the younger brothers died of AIDS; his family later claimed that the monastery had suppressed news of his illness and had prevented him from seeking proper treatment out of fear of public scandal. Although the lawsuit was eventually settled out of court with a minimum of publicity, the incident brought into the open some long-simmering concerns among the monks about the style of leadership practiced at the monastery, as well as unresolved conflicts about celibacy, sexuality, and homophobia in the modern church.

On the other hand, some communities are quite open about their factions and gladly accept the conflicts that may ensue when opposing groups contend for political, economic, or social resources. In Trinidad, for example, there are multiple levels at which political factionalism (usually rooted in racial and/or ethnic divisions) affects the way people go about their lives. Among the Indians, there are divisions between Hindus and Muslims, while in a larger sense there is an often bitter rivalry between Indians as a group and "creoles" as a group. The major national political parties have tended to represent one or another of these general factors—the rare experiments in pluralistic parties have not lasted for very long. Even in A.A., there was a drawn-out battle between those who insisted on strict adherence to "the Big Book" (the tenets of treatment originally developed by the legendary Bill W. back in the 1930s) and those who sought to modify those principles in light of the realities of Trinidadian society and Indian culture. Fieldworkers cannot help but be entangled in these disputes simply by virtue of their being on the scene and striving to become active participants in the life of the community; that life includes factionalism, and researchers are expected to take sides. If they choose to do so, they must acknowledge the probability of the other side withholding further cooperation; if they choose not to do so, they must be very careful in explaining to everyone why being even-handed does not mean indifference to matters of profound concern to people in the community.

Evaluating Tales from the Field

In light of the apparent break-down of the once-unchallenged, authoritative voice of field researchers who knew things their audiences could not because, after all, they were *there*, how can we judge the worth of ethnographic accounts? If "reality" is socially constructed, and if there are multiple voices by which "truth" may be spoken, does it even make sense to seek ways to determine accuracy? By what standards can we say that reports of field observations are convincing? We have already seen how qualitative researchers in general have modified the quantitative concepts of validity and reliability. If those measures of assessment are set aside, are we left with nothing more than the feeling that one set of observations is just as good as any other?

Relativism and the evaluation of field research.

Most researchers are uncomfortable embracing relativism to the extent that all assessments are thrown out. There is some agreement that "ethnography has a distinctive capacity to make discoveries about the social world that had been unknown or misknown," suggesting that it would be a mistake to conclude that "anything goes" (Emerson, 2001, p. 296). It is therefore necessary to come up with criteria that help us evaluate ethnographic research which are sensitive to a constructivist view of reality, even as they make critical distinctions in assessing the quality of accounts derived from that research.

One approach relies on a strategy of **member validation**. The obvious connotation of this term is that researchers must submit their findings to the people they studied; if the members agree that it is accurate, then the external audience for the research could have confidence in the resulting report (Douglas, 1976). This strategy sounds like a good idea, but it often founders in practice. After all, it is probably not possible to satisfy *every* member of even a small group; how do we know how to constitute an adequate representative sample?

On a more conceptual level, is it *always* appropriate to give priority to the emic over the etic interpretation of human behavior? Perhaps in response to these reservations, a secondary meaning of "member validation" has been developed; it involves a test of whether an ethnographic account in and of itself is adequate to provide an outsider with sufficient information to "pass" as an

insider (Wiseman, 1970). This standard, however, relies on the feasibility of conducting some sort of controlled "naturalistic experiment," something not always easy to carry off, and not always amenable to unambiguous interpretation. It also relies on the assumption that a richly detailed account is automatically more useful than a thin description; the former may be the product of a skilled ethnographic writer, not necessarily of a skilled fieldworker.

Another approach to evaluation involves the use of the criterion of **theoretical originality**. A study could be deemed a success either by making a demonstrable contribution to an existing body of theory or developing a new theoretical synthesis of its own (Hammersley, 1992). Quite aside from the fact that at least some researchers are not really interested in theory in any formal way (there still being an honored place in ethnography for purely descriptive studies that contribute mainly on the substantive level), there is the problem that this approach simply reverses the problem with member validation by prioritizing the etic over the "emic." In effect, is "reality" what members of the community (with their admittedly limited view) think it is, or what informed (but inexperienced) outsiders think it is?

A related theoretical concern centers on the concept of **transferability**, the degree to which the findings of the case under study can be shown to be similar to other cases (Lincoln and Guba, 1985: 296–298). This principle differs from "generalizability," which is predicated on making statements that are held to be true in a general sense. With transferability, it is only necessary to demonstrate that one case is similar to another. Adhering strictly to this principle, however, begs the question: is a truly unique case (if such a thing exists) therefore necessarily to be rejected?

Yet another approach to the evaluation of field observations is through the careful explication of research methods. It used to be common in anthropology, for example, for an ethnographer to toss off a phrase to the effect that "I collected data by means of participant observation," and assume that readers would understand. Nowadays, a careful, step-by-step review of the procedures of fieldwork is considered to be absolutely critical if an analysis of a field account is to be taken at all seriously. Altheide and Johnson (1994, p. 485) refer to this procedure as "validity-as-reflexive accounting."

There are three important facets of any field research project that require particularly careful explication. First, since matters ranging from site selection to focus of observation to choice of observational methods are dependent on researchers' theoretical preferences, it is necessary to make explicit their theoretical orientations so that their audiences can evaluate the research. Knowing the theoretical orientation helps the audience understand why certain choices were made in the course of doing the fieldwork and analyzing the resulting data. Second, the ethnographer must discuss clearly and completely the ways in which relations with people in the field were initiated and maintained. In other words, it is necessary to discuss the role adopted by the researcher, the reasons for that choice, and the implications of assuming that role for the conduct of research. Finally, it is necessary to explain the "analytic assumptions and interpretive devices used to collect, interpret, and organize field data" (Emerson, 2001, p. 305).

In sum, if the audience has a clear understanding of how the researcher conceived of, carried out, and made final sense of the project, then it is in a better position to say whether or not the study is convincing. One final note of caution, however: the principle of validity-as-reflexive-accounting can give the audience some confidence that researchers know what they are doing, which is not at all the same thing as concluding that their account in any way represents "reality." The vexing issue thus remains: Is there any way to express confidence in ethnographic accounts without at the same time falling into the old habit of assuming that there is an objective reality "out there," and that it is the sole task of the researcher to capture it faithfully, with a minimum of subjective interpretation?

The principle of verification.

Creswell (1998, p. 200) summarizes the literature on "verification" (a term that might be an appropriate qualitative substitute for "validity," which has too many affinities to quantitative inquiry) and concludes that there are four main themes: some researchers (e.g., LeCompte and Goetz, 1982) insist on standards that are parallel to those of quantitative research so that qualitative findings are readily acceptable to quantifiers; others (e.g., Eisner, 1991; Lincoln and Guba, 1985) suggest developing alternate terms that recognize the distinctive characteristics of naturalistic field research; still others (e.g., Lather, 1993; Richardson, 1990) advocate a complete reconceptualization of the concept in light of postmodernist perspectives on "reality"; and another contingent (e.g., Wolcott, 1994) believe that the whole discussion is simply

irrelevant to doing good ethnographic work and that the search for appropriate ways to validate, verify, or otherwise evaluate qualitative research is an unnecessary distraction. A possibly useful compromise was suggested by Spindler and Spindler (1987) who proposed a set of standards for a "good ethnography. Their list includes the following:

- Be sure that all observations are placed in their fullest possible context when they are used in a report about field research. In effect, actions and interactions do not occur in a vacuum; they happen in specific places at specific times and under specific circumstances. But as observations are repeated, it becomes possible to sort of patterns of regularity from behaviors that are temporary or random.

- Be sure that the insiders' perspective is obtained. It need not be the final determinant of what is "real," but internal meanings can never be discarded simply for the sake of reaching broad, general conclusions.

- Any other kinds of data collection (e.g., interviews, questionnaires) should flow from observations made on site, and not be composed beforehand and inserted without modification in a particular setting.

It is the job of the field researcher to make explicit what is implicit and tacit to members of the study community. It is also possible to treat verification as a matter of procedures that serve to build an audience's confidence in the trustworthiness of a report from the field. Some of these procedures (e.g., triangulation, repeated observations, member validation, thick description) have been discussed in other contexts. To that list Creswell (1998, pp. 201–203) adds the following:

- **Peer review** (**debriefing**) is a process by which another researcher (presumably one who has not been involved in the project at hand) plays "devil's advocate" by asking hard questions about methods, meanings, and interpretations.

- **Negative case analysis** entails the progressive refinement of working hypotheses or research questions in light of negative or disconfirming evidence that crops up in the course of the research. The questions are revised until all cases fit and all seeming outliers and exceptions are accounted for.

- **External audits** involve an external consultant who assesses the product of research and comes to a conclusion about whether or not the findings, interpretations, and conclusions are supported by the data. This procedure differs from the peer review in that it is not a dialogue about a work in process; the audit is applied only to a product that has already been completed.

Creswell (1998, p. 203) recommends that researchers apply at least two of these procedures in any given project.

For Discussion

1. Consider your own proposed research project. Select any one of the issues discussed in this chapter and write a reflective essay commenting on how you might re-think your proposal in light of this discussion.

2. Consider the published study you have been working with. In what way does any one of the issues discussed in this chapter play a role in helping you understand how the study was conducted and presented?

Chapter Seven

Looking Ahead

It seems safe to say that observation will continue to be an essential element in the tool kit of qualitative field researchers. Despite the controversial questions discussed in the previous section, we will continue to make detailed, systematic observations of one form or another are the foundation for everything else we do in our study of human groups in their natural settings. It can be taken as a given that "forecasting the wax and wane of social science research methods is always uncertain" (Adler and Adler, 1994, p. 389), but it is still possible to venture some guesses as to what might be in the near future for observational techniques.

First, it is very likely that observational research will become increasingly committed to "the ethnography of the particular" (Abu-Lughod, 1991, p. 154). Most of the research traditions that gave rise to and sustained observational methods aimed to describe presumably homogeneous, coherent, patterned, and timeless nature of the group. They sought to discern the composite culture of a group (e.g., historical particularism) or to analyze the full range of institutions that constituted the society (e.g., functionalism). The "ethnography of the particular," by contrast, seeks to provide a rounded account of the lives of particular people, emphasizing the ever-changing relationships with which individuals are involved. This shift in emphasis will impact not only the traditional social science disciplines (anthropology, sociology, social psychology), but may also effect a change in such hybrid fields as "cultural studies," which may have to move away from their focus on the abstract and the presumably general and bring their theoretical constructs down to the level of everyday behavior.

Observation could, until fairly recently, be carried out with a notebook, pencil, sketch pad, and perhaps a simple tape recorder and camera. The conduct of observational research was revitalized by the introduction of video recording technology while even basic functions such as note-taking and pattern-finding have been transformed by the advent of laptop computers and data-analysis software. These technical advances, while beneficial for the most part, do raise an interesting dilemma. On the one hand, we have come to embrace the theoretical language of "situatedness," indeterminacy, and relativism. But on the other hand, advanced technology gives us the illusion that we are in a better position than ever to capture "reality." That technology

makes it possible for us to record and analyze people and events with a degree of particularity that would have been unthinkable just a few years ago; but the apparently unchallengeable accuracy of new recording media threaten to privilege whatever is captured on tape (audio or visual) over the lived experience of ethnographers. In the early twentieth century, a fieldworker could say, "Believe me—I was there and you were not." Nowadays, one might well say, "Believe me—and here's the video to prove it." But as we have seen in the previous section, even the most acutely calibrated recording devices record only what a fieldworker chooses to record; and all recording media necessarily include capabilities for editing. Our culture's fascination with technology as an absolute standard thus runs counter to what we have learned—at great intellectual expense—about the multivocalic, ever-changing nature of social "reality." It might therefore become necessary for us to turn an increasingly critical eye on our methods—not only to explicate the how-to's, but also to examine the (often unspoken) philosophical assumptions that support our methods.

As Postman (1993) and other students of communication have pointed out, technological change is never simply additive; that is, is does not merely allow us to do the same old things, only more efficiently. Rather, it is "ecological," in the sense that a change in one aspect of behavior has ramifications for the entire system of which that behavior is a part. (This perception, by the way, is an interesting latter-day take on the old functionalist paradigm that understood societies as if they were organic systems; in order to maintain a semblance of equilibrium, change in one institution necessitated compensatory changes in all the others to which it was connected.) Technology, in other words, is not simply an adjunct to business-as-usual; it becomes a defining quality of our culture as researchers. As such, we might do well to devote more of our energies to studying ourselves as we study others (Tedlock, 2005). In other words, we need to turn our observational skills on the encounters we ourselves create; we must observe not only what happens when "we" encounter "them," but also what happens to us when we mediate those encounters via a particular kind of technology that has the capacity to transform both our way of seeing and our way of understanding the world.

Ethics Revisited

In the near term, we will almost certainly continue to grapple with the ethical ramifications of our research. A recent report from the Institute of Medicine (IOM)—a body that one would think would represent an old, established paradigm of research ethics—challenged researchers in all disciplines to rethink the whole notion of research ethics. The IOM report pointed out that we have become used to asking basically negative questions (e.g., what is misconduct? how can it be prevented?). It might be preferable to consider the positive and ask, what is integrity? how do we find out whether we have it? how can we encourage it? The promotion of researcher integrity has both individual and institutional components, and those in charge of monitoring professional ethics should be in the business of "encouraging individuals to be intellectually honest in their work and to act responsibly, and encouraging research institutions to provide an environment in which that behavior can thrive" (Grinnell, 2002, p. B15). A re-thought IRB might well function with something more than a utilitarian checklist of presumed (negative) consequences. It could instead constitute a circle of "wise peers" (Gula, 1989, p. 278) with whom researchers could discuss and work out the sometimes conflicting demands of experience, intuition, and the potential for rational analysis and argument. The essential problem with current ethical codes, according to the IOM (and a position that I believe most qualitative observational researchers would endorse) is that they set up an arbitrary and unnecessary adversarial relationship between researchers and the rest of the scholarly community. The IOM went so far as to suggest that qualitative social researchers have a central role to play in this proposed evolution of the structures of research ethics because they are particularly well equipped to conduct studies that could identify and assess the factors influencing integrity in research in both individuals and large social institutions.

I would like to close with a quote from the late Stephen Jay Gould (1998, p. 72), the renowned paleontologist and historian of science, that I have cited in other of my writings on the observational method. To my mind it is instructive that this exemplar of the scientific method should conclude the following:

No faith can be more misleading than an unquestioned personal conviction that the apparent testimony of one's eyes must provide a purely objective account, scarcely requiring any validation beyond the claim itself. Utterly unbiased observation must rank as a primary myth and shibboleth of science, for we can only see what fits into our mental space, and all description includes interpretation as well as sensory reporting.

Glossary

Archival Research

The study of culture and society through documentary records

Behavior Trace Studies

The use of artifacts left behind in the wake of human activity in order to conduct an indirect study of that activity

Census

A descriptive listing of every person, household unit, or any other thing important in a study community

Content Analysis

The study of formal texts as clues to social and cultural behavior

Continuous Monitoring

Observations conducted over a designated period of time, with behaviors recorded in minute detail

Counting

The enumeration of types of people, material items, locations, or other things that are important for situating an event, location, or activity in its proper community context

Cultural Relativism

A principle that treats behaviors in their proper cultural contexts, avoiding judgments about their merits

Culture Shock

A feeling of uncertainty and dislocation experienced by field researchers as they adjust to a setting in which familiar cues may be absent

Debriefing

see **Peer Review**

Deductive Inquiry

A research process that begins with general propositions and works down to specific illustrative examples

Descriptive Analysis

The process of breaking down a body of data into its component parts to see if there are any discernable regularities, patterns, or themes

Disguised Observations

Research carried out by researchers who blend thoroughly into their study populations and whose conduct of research is not apparent to anyone else in the setting

Emic Analysis

The explication of social and cultural patterns, regularities, and themes as they are understood by people in a study community

Ethnicity

A social category based
on shared culture

Ethnocentrism

The tendency to think that the way
of doing and thinking about things
that is typical or one's own culture is
inherently the best and most logical

Ethnography

The descriptive study of people
in their natural settings

Ethnomethodology

A school of sociological and
social psychological theory that
is primarily concerned with
how people construct order
in their groups

Etic Analysis

The explication of social and cultural
patterns, regularities and themes as
they are perceived by the outside
researcher operating from a cross-
culturally comparative point of view

External Audit

A verification procedure,
entailing a process whereby an
expert not involved in a research
project assesses the research product
and comes to a conclusion
about whether the findings,
interpretations, and conclusions
are supported by the data

Fieldwork

Any form of research conducted in a
natural setting as opposed to a
controlled laboratory or clinical
setting

Flowchart

A diagram depicting the movement
of people, products, or behaviors
through a sequence of events

Functionalism

A school of anthropological
and sociological theory that
conceptualizes society as a system
of institutions that operate together
in order to achieve overall
balance and equilibrium

Gatekeepers

People who, officially or unofficially,
control access to a study population

Gender

The set of behaviors and other
learned characteristics that are
considered to be culturally
appropriate manifestations
of a person's biological sex

Hierarchical Tree

A diagram showing different levels of
abstraction in a theoretical analysis

Historical Particularism

A school of anthropological theory
emphasizing the distinctive process
of change that characterizes each
culture

Inductive Inquiry

A research process that begins with
specific empirical observations and
builds toward general propositions

Informed Consent
A principle of ethical research that requires potential study participants to be fully informed about the procedures and expected outcomes of the project and to give their formal agreement to being observed or otherwise studied

Key Informants
Persons who have specialized knowledge about selected aspects of life in a study community

Matrix
A table comparing two or more segments of a study population in terms of a selected analytic category

Member Validation
A verification procedure entailing the presentation of research findings to members of the study community to test the accuracy of the account alternatively, a test of whether an ethnographic account is in and of itself sufficiently informative to allow an outsider to "pass" as a member of the study community

Metaphors
Literary figures of speech used to express the quality of relationships

Naturalistic Field Experiments
A situation created or manipulated by researchers in order to result in behavior that can be observed and analyzed

Negative Case Analysis
A verification procedure entailing the progressive refinement of working hypotheses or research questions in light of negative or disconfirming evidence that comes up in the course of research questions are revised until all cases fit and all seeming outliers and exceptions are accounted for

Non-Reactive Observation
see **Unobtrusive Observation**

Observation
In qualitative research, the study of people interacting in their natural settings so that their behaviors and words can be put into their proper context

Organizational Chart
A diagram depicting the relationship of elements within a structured system

Participant Observation
Study undertaken by a researcher who strives to be an active member of the group being observed

Peer Review
A verification procedure entailing a process by which a researcher not involved in a given project engages the person who actually conducted the project in a dialogue about methods, meanings, and interpretations

Public Space
A setting that is open and that requires no special permission to access for purposes of research

Qualitative Research

A process of inquiry that aims to understand human behavior by building complex, holistic pictures of the social and cultural settings in which such behavior occurs

Race

A social category based on presumed biological affinities

Reactive Observation

The study of human behavior by researchers who are identified as such, but are not otherwise considered members of the study community

Reflexive Narratives

Representations of field data that incorporate a subjective understanding of the experiences of the people in the subject community and that are told in such a way as to incorporate reflections by the researcher on the experience of conducting the study

Reliability

A measure of the degree to which there is consistency in the research process

Social Indicators

Material artifacts or other conditions that can be used to demarcate differences among groups within a study community

Social Research

Inquiry into the nature of social institutions and/or of the patterns of belief and customary behavior that form the cultural core of those institutions

Spot Sampling

Observations conducted at randomly selected places, at randomly selected times in order to record a sufficiently large number of representative acts

Structured Observation

see **Reactive Observation**

Studying Up

Conducting research among social elites or in the institutions that control disadvantaged populations

Symbolic Interactionism

A school of sociological and social psychological theory that treats society as the ever-changing product of negotiated interactions among participants

Systematic Research

Inquiry that is conducted carefully, with precise notation that allows for the efficient retrieval of information and the orderly categorization and analysis of that information

Theoretical Analysis

The process of explaining why perceived regularities, patterns, or themes exist in a body of data

Time Allocation

see **Spot Sampling**

Transferability

A criterion of verification involving the degree to which the findings of one case study can be shown to be similar to the conditions pertaining to one or more other cases

Thick Description

A way of looking at a setting or event as it might be seen through the eyes of those participating in it so as to discern the structures of meaning through which people produce, perceive, and interpret their own and others' activities

Triangulation

The use of multiple data collection techniques and data sources in order to converge on a comprehensive account of a field setting

Unobtrusive Observation

Study undertaken by a researcher who avoids intervening in the action being observed

Validity

A measure of the degree to which research findings conform to objective reality

Verification

A qualitative analog to the more quantifiable principle of validity

Verstehen

The subjective understanding of what people in a study community are doing

Virtual Communities

Groups formed on-line by people sharing some defined common interest

Vulnerable Populations

Groups of people defined in the standards of ethical research as being particularly at risk of physical or psychological harm when involved in research projects

References

Abu-Lughod, L. (1991). Writing against culture. In R. G. Fox (Ed.), *Recapturing anthropology: Working in the present* (pp. 137–162). Santa Fe, NM: School of American Research.

Adler, P. A., & Adler, P. (1994). Observational techniques. In N. K. Denzin & Y. S. Lincoln (Eds.), *Handbook of qualitative research* (pp. 377–392). Thousand Oaks, CA: Sage.

Agar, M. (1980). *The professional stranger: An informal introduction to ethnography.* San Diego, CA: Academic Press.

Albrecht, G. L. (1985). Videotape safaris: entering the field with a camera. *Qualitative Sociology, 8,* 325–344.

Altheide, D. L., & Johnson, J. M. (1994). Criteria for assessing interpretive validity in qualitative research. In N. K. Denzin & Y. S. Lincoln (Eds.), *Handbook of qualitative research* (pp. 485–499). Thousand Oaks, CA: Sage.

Altork, K. (1995). Walking the fire line: the erotic dimension of the fieldwork experience. In D. Kulick & M. Willson (Eds.), *Taboo: Sex, identity and erotic subjectivity in anthropological fieldwork* (pp. 107–139). London: Routledge.

Angrosino, M. V. (1974). *Outside is death.* Winston-Salem, NC: Medical Behavioral Sciences Monograph Series.

Angrosino, M. V. (1997). Among the savage anthros: Reflections on the SAS oral history project. *Southern Anthropologist, 24,* 98–109.

Angrosino, M. V. (1998a). Mental disability in the United States: An interactionist perspective. In R. Jenkins (Ed.), *Questions of competence: Culture, classification and intellectual disability* (pp. 25–53). Cambridge, UK: Cambridge University Press.

Angrosino, M. V. (1998b). *Opportunity House: Ethnographic stories of mental retardation.* Walnut Creek, CA: AltaMira.

Angrosino, M. V. (2004). Disclosure and interaction in a monastery. In
L. Hume & J. Mulcock (Eds.), *Anthropologists in the field: Cases in
participant observation* (pp. 18–32). New York: Columbia University
Press.

Angrosino, M. V. (2006). *Blessed with enough foolishness: Pastoral care
in a modern hospital.* West Conshohocken, PA: Infinity Press.

Atkinson, P. A. (1990). *The ethnographic imagination: Textual constructions
of reality.* London: Routledge.

Atkinson, P. A. (1992). *Understanding ethnographic texts.*
Newbury Park, CA: Sage.

Behar, R. (1993). *Translated woman: Crossing the border with
Esperanza's story.* Boston: Beacon.

Belo, J. (1960). *Trance in Bali.* New York: Columbia University Press.

Berg, B. L. (2004). *Qualitative research methods for the social sciences*
(5th ed.). Boston: Pearson.

Berger, L., & Ellis, C. (2002). Composing autoethnographic stories. In M. V.
Angrosino (Ed.), *Doing cultural anthropology: Projects for ethnographic
data collection* (pp. 151–166). Prospect Heights, IL: Waveland.

Bernard, H. R. (1988). *Research methods in cultural anthropology.*
Newbury Park, CA: Sage.

Bird, S. E. (2003). *The audience in everyday life: Living in a media world.*
New York: Routledge.

Bittner, E. (1973). Objectivity and realism in sociology. In G. Psathas (Ed.),
Phenomenological sociology: Issues and applications (pp. 109–125).
New York: Wiley.

Blackwood, E. (1995). Falling in love with an-Other lesbian: Reflections
on identity in fieldwork. In D. Kulick & M. Willson (Eds.), *Taboo: Sex,
identity and erotic subjectivity in anthropological fieldwork* (pp. 51–75).
London: Routledge

Borman, K., Puccia, E., McNulty, A. F., & Goddard, B. (2002). Observing a workplace. In M. V. Angrosino (Ed.), *Doing cultural anthropology: Projects for ethnographic data collection* (pp. 99–106). Prospect Heights, IL: Waveland.

Bottorff, J. L. (1994). Using videotaped recordings in qualitative research. In J. M. Morse (Ed.), *Critical issues in qualitative research methods* (pp. 244–261). Thousand Oaks, CA: Sage.

Bourgois, P. (2002). Workaday world, crack economy. In J. H. McDonald (Ed.), *The applied anthropology reader* (pp. 149–156). Boston: Allyn & Bacon.

Buchanan, E. A. (Ed.). (2004). *Readings in virtual research ethics: Issues and controversies*. Hershey, PA: Information Sciences Publishing.

Cahill, S. E. (2004). The interaction order of public bathrooms. In S. E. Cahill (Ed.), *Inside social life: Readings in sociological psychology and microsociology* (4th ed., pp. 167–177). Los Angeles: Roxbury.

Casagrande, J. (Ed.). (1960). *In the company of man*. New York: Harper Brothers.

Chambers, E. (2000). Applied ethnography. In N. K. Denzin & Y. S. Lincoln (Eds.), *Handbook of qualitative research* (2nd ed., pp. 851–869). Thousand Oaks, CA: Sage.

Clark, L., & Werner, O. (1997). Protection of human subjects and ethnographic photography. *Cultural Anthropology Methods, 9(3)*, 18–20.

Clifford, J. (1997). Spatial practices: Fieldwork, travel, and the disciplining of anthropology. In A. Gupta & J. Ferguson (Eds.), *Anthropological locations: Boundaries and grounds for a field science* (pp. 185–222). Berkeley: University of California Press.

Collier, J. (1967). *Visual anthropology: Photography as a research method*. New York: Holt, Rinehart & Winston.

Creswell, J. W. (1998). *Qualitative inquiry and research design: Choosing among five traditions*. Thousand Oaks, CA: Sage.

Dalla, R. L. (2000). Exposing the 'Pretty Woman' myth: A qualitative exposition of the lives of female streetwalking prostitutes. *Journal of Sex Research, 37(4)*, 344–353.

Diamond, J. (2003). Race without color. In A. Podolefsky & P. J. Brown (Eds.), *Applying anthropology: An introductory reader* (pp. 203–209). Boston: McGraw Hill.

Douglas, J. D. (1976). *Investigative social research: Individual and team field research.* Beverly Hills, CA: Sage.

Duneier, M. (1994). *Sidewalk.* New York: Farrar, Straus and Giroux.

Eisner, E. W. (1991). *The enlightened eye: Qualitative inquiry and the enhancement of educational practice.* New York: Macmillan.

Elliott, D., & Stern, J.E. (Eds.). (1997). *Research ethics: A reader.* Hanover, NH: University Press of New England.

Ellis, C. (1995). *Final negotiations: A story of love, loss, and chronic illness.* Philadelphia: Temple University Press.

Ellis, C., & Bochner, A. P. (2000). Autoethnography, personal narrative, reflexivity: Researcher as subject. In N. K. Denzin & Y. S. Lincoln (Eds.) *Handbook of qualitative research* (2nd ed., pp. 733–768). Newbury Park, CA: Sage.

Emerson, R. M. (2001). *Contemporary field research: Perspectives and formulations* (2nd ed.). Prospect Heights, IL: Waveland.

Fassnacht, G. (1982). *Theory and practice of observing behavior.* New York: Academic Press.

Fetterman, D. M. (1998). *Ethnography: Step by step* (2nd ed.). Thousand Oaks, CA: Sage.

Fluehr-Lobban, C. (Ed.). (2003). *Ethics and the profession of anthropology: Dialogue for ethically conscious practice* (2nd ed.). Walnut Creek, CA: AltaMira.

Freeman, L., Romney, A. K., & Freeman, S. C. (1987). Cognitive structure and informant accuracy. *American Anthropologist, 89,* 310–325.

Gearing, J. (1995). Fear and loving in the West Indies: Research from the heart (as well as the head). In D. Kulick & M. Willson (Eds.), *Taboo: Sex, identity and erotic subjectivity in anthropological fieldwork* (pp. 186–218). London: Routledge.

Geertz, C. (1973). *The interpretation of cultures.* New York: Basic Books.

Gold, R. L. (1958). Roles in sociological field observations. *Social Forces, 36,* 217–223.

Gould, R. A., & Potter, P. B. (1984). *Use-lives of automobiles in America: A preliminary archaeological view.* Providence, RI: Research Papers in Anthropology, Department of Anthropology, Brown University.

Gould, S. J. (1998). The sharp-eyed lynx, outfoxed by nature (part 2). *Natural History 107,* 23–27, 69–73.

Gouldner, A. W. (1962). Anti-minotaur: The myth of a value-free sociology. *Social Problems, 9,* 199–213.

Grindal, B. T., & Salamone, F. A. (Eds.). (2006). *Bridges to humanity: Narratives on fieldwork and friendship* (2nd ed.). Long Grove, IL: Waveland.

Grinnell, F. (2002). *The impact of ethics on research.* Washington, DC: Institute of Medicine.

Gruenbaum, E. (2001). *The female circumcision controversy: An anthropological perspective.* Philadelphia: University of Pennsylvania Press.

Gubrium, J. F., & Holstein, J. A. (1997). *The new language of qualitative methods.* New York: Oxford University Press.

Guilmet, G. M. (1979). Instructor reaction to verbal and nonverbal-visual behavior in the urban classroom. *Anthropology and Education Quarterly, 10,* 254–266.

Gula, R. M. (1989). *Reason informed by faith.* New York: Paulist Press.

Gupta, A., & Ferguson, J. (1997). Discipline and practice: 'The field' as site, method, and location in anthropology. In A. Gupta & J. Ferguson (Eds.), *Anthropological locations: Boundaries and grounds for a field science* (pp. 1–46). Berkeley: University of California Press.

Gwynne, M. A. (2003). *Applied anthropology: A career-oriented approach.* Boston: Pearson.

Hakken, D. (2003). An ethics for an anthropology in and of cyberspace. In C. Fluehr-Lobban (Ed.), *Ethics and the profession of anthropology: Dialogue for ethically conscious practice* (2nd ed., pp. 179–195). Walnut Creek, CA: AltaMira.

Hall, E. T. (1966). *The hidden dimension.* New York: Doubleday.

Hammersley, M. (1992). *What's wrong with ethnography? Methodological explorations.* London: Routledge.

Haraway, D. (1998). Situated knowledges: The science question in feminism and the privilege of partial perspective. *Feminist Studies, 14,* 575–599.

Heath, S. B. (1983). *Ways with words: Language, life, and work in communities and classrooms.* New York: Cambridge University Press.

Heider, K. (1976). *Ethnographic film.* Austin: University of Texas Press.

Herman-Kinney, N. J., & Verschaeve, J. M (2003). Methods of symbolic interaction. In L. T. Reynolds & N. J. Herman-Kinney (Eds.), *Handbook of symbolic interactionism* (pp. 213–252). Walnut Creek, CA: AltaMira.

Holstein, J. A., & Gubrium, J. F. (1994). Phenomenology, ethnomethodology, and interpretive practice. In N. K. Denzin & Y. S. Lincoln (Eds.), *Handbook of qualitative research* (pp. 262–272). Thousand Oaks, CA: Sage.

Holmes, L. D. (1986). *Quest for the real Samoa: The Mead/Freeman controversy and beyond.* South Hadley, MA: Bergin & Garvey.

Hume, L., & Mulcock, J. (Eds.). (2004). *Anthropologists in the field: Cases in participant observation.* New York: Columbia University Press.

Humphreys, L. (1975). *Tearoom trade: Impersonal sex in public places.* Chicago: Aldine.

Johnson, A. (1975). Time allocation in a Machiguenga community. *Ethnology, 14,* 310–321.

Kirk, J., & Miller, M. L. (1986). *Reliability and validity in qualitative research.* Beverly Hills, CA: Sage.

Kottak, C. P., & Kozaitis, K. A. (2003). *On being different: Diversity and multiculturalism in the North American mainstream* (2nd ed.). Boston: McGraw-Hill.

Kulick, D., & Willson, M. (Eds.). (1995). *Taboo: Sex, identity and erotic subjectivity in anthropological fieldwork.* London: Routledge.

Lally, E. F. (2006). State-of-the-art digital cameras. *Anthropology News, 47*(9), 24.

Lang, S. (1996). Traveling woman: Conducting a fieldwork project on gender variance and homosexuality among North American Indians. In E. Lewin & W. Leap (Eds.), *Out in the field: Reflections of lesbian and gay anthropologists* (pp. 86–110). Urbana: University of Illinois Press.

Lather, P. (1993). Fertile obsession: Validity after poststructuralism. *Sociological Quarterly, 34,* 673–693.

Le Compte, M. D., & Goetz, J. P. (1982). Problems of reliability and validity in ethnographic research. *Review of Educational Research, 51,* 31–60.

Lee, R. B. (1969). A naturalist at large: Eating Christmas in the Kalahari. *Natural History, 78,* 14–22, 60–64.

Lee, R. B.. & De Vore, I. (1969). *Man the hunter.* Chicago: Aldine.

Lehner, P. N. (1979). *Handbook of ethological methods.* New York: Garland STPM.

Lewin, E., & Leap, W. L. (Eds.). (1996). *Out in the field: Reflections of lesbian and gay anthropologists.* Urbana: University of Illinois Press.

Liazos, A. (1972). The poverty of the sociology of deviance: Nuts, sluts, and perverts. *Social Problems, 20,* 103–20.

Liebow, E. (1967). *Tally's corner: A study of Negro streetcorner men.* Boston: Little, Brown.

Lincoln, Y. S. (2005). Institutional review boards and methodological conservatism: The challenge to and from phenomenological paradigms. In N. K. Denzin & Y. S. Lincoln (Eds.), *Handbook of qualitative research* (3rd ed., pp. 165–182). Thousand Oaks, CA: Sage.

Lincoln, Y. S., & Denzin, N. K. (Eds.). (2003). *Turning points in qualitative research: Tying knots in a handkerchief.* Walnut Creek, CA: AltaMira.

Lincoln, Y. S., & Guba, E. (1985). *Naturalistic inquiry.* Beverly Hills, CA: Sage.

Lipson, J. G. (1994). Ethical issues in ethnography. In J. M. Morse (Ed.), *Critical issues in qualitative research methods* (pp. 333–355). Thousand Oaks, CA: Sage.

Malkki, L. H. (1996). News and culture: Transitory phenomena and the fieldwork tradition. In A. Gupta & J. Ferguson (Eds.), *Culture, power, place: Explorations in critical anthropology* (pp. 86–101). Durham, NC: Duke University Press.

Markham, A. N. (2005). The methods, politics, and ethics of representation in online ethnography. In N. K. Denzin & Y. S. Lincoln (Eds.), *Handbook of qualitative research* (3rd ed., pp. 793–820). Thousand Oaks, CA: Sage.

McGee, R. J., & Warms, R. L. (2004). *Anthropological theory: An introductory history* (3rd ed.). Boston: McGraw Hill.

Mead, M., & Bateson, G. (1977). On the use of the camera in anthropology. *Studies in the Anthropology of Visual Communication, 4,* 78–80.

Mienczakowski, J. (1996). The ethnographic act. In C. Ellis & A. Bochner (Eds.), *Composing ethnography: Alternative forms of qualitative writing* (pp. 244–264). Walnut Creek, CA: AltaMira.

Milgram, S. (1963). Behavioral studies of obedience. *Journal of Abnormal and Social Psychology, 67,* 371–378.

Miller, D., & Slater, D. (2000). *The internet: An ethnographic approach.* New York: Berg.

Moreno, E. (1995). Rape in the field: Reflections from a survivor. In D. Kulick & M. Willson (Eds.), *Taboo: Sex, identity and erotic subjectivity in anthropological fieldwork* (pp. 219–250). London: Routledge.

Nader, L. (1969). Up the anthropologist—perspectives gained from studying up. In D. Hymes (Ed.), *Reinventing anthropology* (pp. 284–311). New York: Vintage.

Niebel, B. W. (1982). *Motion and time study* (7th ed.). Homewood, IL: Irwin.

Oboler, R. W. (1985). *Women, power, and economic change: The Nandi of Kenya*. Stanford, CA: Stanford University Press.

Poehlman, J. A. (2004). *Community participation and consensus in HIV/AIDS prevention*. Unpublished doctoral dissertation, University of South Florida.

Postman, N. (1993). *Technopoly: The surrender of culture to technology*. New York: Vintage.

Price, L. J. (2002). Carrying out a structured observation. In M. V. Angrosino (Ed.), *Doing cultural anthropology: Projects for ethnographic data collection* (pp. 107–114). Prospect Heights, IL: Waveland.

Punch, M. (1986). *The politics and ethics of fieldwork*. Beverly Hills, CA: Sage.

Rathje, W. L. (1984). The garbage decade. *American Behavioral Scientist, 28*, 9–29.

Redfern-Vance, N. (1999). *Narratives of women veterans: The experience of sexual abuse*. Unpublished doctoral dissertation, University of South Florida.

Richardson, L. (1990). *Writing strategies: Reaching diverse audiences*. Newbury Park, CA: Sage.

Richardson, L. (1992). The consequences of poetic representation. In C. Ellis & M. Flaherty (Eds.), *Investigating subjectivity* (pp. 125–140). Newbury Park, CA: Sage.

Riessman, C. K. (1987). When gender is not enough: Women interviewing women. *Gender and Society, 1*, 172–207.

Schensul, S. L., Schensul, J. J., & LeCompte, M. D. (1999). *Essential ethnographic methods: Observations, interviews, and questionnaires*. Walnut Creek, CA: AltaMira.

Sechrest, L., & Flores, L. (1969). Homosexuality in the Philippines and the United States: The handwriting on the wall. *Journal of Social Psychology, 79*, 3–12.

Smith, L. T. (2005). On tricky ground: Researching the native in the age of uncertainty. In N. K. Denzin & Y. S. Lincoln (Eds.), *Handbook of qualitative research* (3rd ed., pp. 85–107). Thousand Oaks, CA: Sage.

Sparkes, A. C. (2002). *Telling tales in sport and physical activity: A qualitative journey.* Champaign, IL: Human Kinetics.

Spindler, G., & Spindler, L. (1987). Teaching and learning how to do the ethnography of education. In G. Spindler & L. Spindler (Eds.), *Interpretive ethnography of education: At home and abroad* (pp. 17–33). Hillsdale, NJ: Lawrence Erlbaum.

Spradley, J. P. (1980). *Participant observation.* New York: Holt, Rinehart and Winston.

Sproull, L. S. (1981). Managing education programs: A micro-behavioral analysis. *Human Organization, 40,* 113–122.

Stocking, G. W. (1983). The ethnographer's magic: Fieldwork in British anthropology from Tylor to Malinowski. In G. W. Stocking (Ed.), *Observers observed: Essays on ethnographic fieldwork* (pp. 70–120). Madison: University of Wisconsin Press.

Sykes, R. E., & Brent, E. E. (1983). *Policing: A social behaviorist perspective.* New Brunswick, NJ: Rutgers University Press.

Tedlock, B. (2005). The observation of participation and the emergence of public ethnography. In N. K. Denzin & Y. S. Lincoln (Eds.), *Handbook of qualitative research* (3rd ed., pp. 467–482). Thousand Oaks, CA: Sage.

Tierney, G. (2002). Becoming a participant observer. In M.V. Angrosino (Ed.), *Doing cultural anthropology: Projects for ethnographic data collection* (pp. 9–18). Prospect Heights, IL: Waveland.

University of Chicago. (2003). *The Chicago manual of style* (15th ed.). Chicago: University of Chicago Press.

Van Maanen, J. (1988). *Tales of the field: On writing ethnography.* Chicago: University of Chicago Press.

Warren, C. A. B. (2001). Gender and fieldwork relations. In R. M. Emerson (Ed.), *Contemporary field research: Perspectives and formulations* (2nd ed., pp. 203–223). Prospect Heights, IL: Waveland.

Webb, E. J., Campbell, D. T., Schwartz, R. C., & Sechrest, L. (1966). *Unobtrusive Measures: Nonreactive Research in the Social Sciences.* Chicago: University of Chicago Press.

Weitzman, E. A., & Miles, M. B. (1995). *Computer programs for qualitative data analysis.* Thousand Oaks, CA: Sage.

Werner, O. & Clark, L. (1998). Ethnographic photographs converted to line drawings. *Cultural Anthropology Methods, 10(3),* 54–56.

Werner, O., & Schoepfle, G. M. (1987). *Systematic fieldwork: Foundations of ethnography and interviewing.* Newbury Park, CA: Sage.

Whitehead, T. L., & Conaway, M. E. (Eds.). (1986). *Self, sex and gender in cross-cultural fieldwork.* Urbana: University of Illinois Press.

Whiting, B. W., & Whiting, J. W. M. (1975). *Children of six cultures: A psycho-cultural analysis.* Cambridge, MA: Harvard University Press.

Wilson, P. J. (1974). *Oscar: An inquiry into the nature of sanity.* New York: Random House.

Wiseman, J. P. (1970). *Stations of the lost: The treatment of Skid Row alcoholics.* Englewood Cliffs, NJ: Prentice-Hall.

Wolcott, H. F. (1994). On seeking—and rejecting—validity in qualitative research. In E. W. Eisner & A. Peshkin (Eds.), *Qualitative inquiry in education: The continuing debate* (pp. 121–152). New York: Columbia University, Teachers College Press.

Wolf, M. A. (1992). *A thrice-told tale: Feminism, postmodernism, and ethnographic responsibility.* Stanford, CA: Stanford University Press.

Zavella, P. (1996). Feminist insider dilemmas: Constructing ethnic identity with 'Chicana' informants. In D. L. Wolfe (Ed.), *Feminist dilemmas in fieldwork* (pp. 138–169). Boulder, CO: Westview.

Zinn, M. B. (1979). Field research in minority communities: Ethical, methodological and political observations by an insider. *Social Problems, 27,* 209–219.

About the Author

Michael V. Angrosino is Professor of Anthropology at the University of South Florida. He has conducted ethnographic fieldwork in the United States and in the West Indies on topics including ethnic identity and cultural diversity, labor migration, mental health policy and service delivery, and the role of organized religion in secular society. He regularly teaches graduate seminars in qualitative methods and oral history. He has contributed major statements on observational research to the *Handbook of Qualitative Research* and the *Encyclopedia of Social Science Research Methods*. He is the co-author of *Field Projects in Anthropology* and the editor of *Doing Cultural Anthropology*, two texts that feature hands-on exercises in conducting ethnographic research. A book on participant observation and a book on oral history methods are both currently in press.

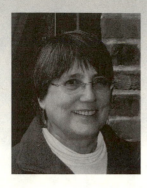

Qualitative Essentials

Series Editor
Janice Morse,
University of Utah

Qualitative Essentials is a book series providing a comprehensive but succinct overview of topics in qualitative inquiry. These books will fill an important niche in qualitative methods for students and others new to qualitative inquiry who require a rapid but complete perspective of specific methods, strategies, and important topics. Written by leaders in qualitative inquiry, alone or in combination, these books will be an excellent resource for instructors and students from all disciplines. Proposals for the series should be sent to the series editor at explore@LCoastPress.com.

Titles from the Qualitative Essentials series:

1. *Naturalistic Observation*, Michael V. Angrosino

Forthcoming Titles:

Qualitative Essentials, Maria Mayan

Focus Groups, Martha Ann Carey

Participatory Action Research, Marilyn Mardiros

Naturalistic
Observation

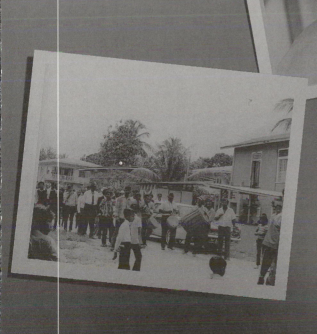